Dr. Abraham C. Knox

VAGUS NERVE EXERCISES

A Practical Guide for Self-Healing Exercises. Learn How to Activate Your Vagus Nerve, Reduce Inflammation, Stop Anxiety, Stress and Chronic Diseases, Depression and PTSD

Real Publishing Press
981, Great West Rd
United Kingdom, Brentford, TW8 9DN
Permissions requests: realpublishing.ltd@gmail.com

Cover Design by Vincent, www.vincentvi.com

Vagus Nerve Exercises / Dr. Abraham C. Knox - First paperback edition
August 2020
ISBN 978-1-913868-02-4

MEDICAL DISCLAIMER: The following information is intended for general information purposes only. Individuals should always see their health care provider before administering any suggestions made in this book. Any application of the material set forth in the following pages is at the reader's discretion and is his or her sole responsibility. The author takes full responsibility for representing and interpreting the ideas related to the Polyvagal Theory. The author's interpretations and representations of the Polyvagal Theory may vary in intent and accuracy from the writings and presentations by Dr. Stephen W. Porges.

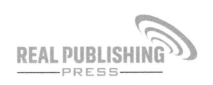

YOUR FREE GIFT

As a way of saying thanks for purchase this book, I'm offering one of our next books for **FREE** to my readers.

Our **VAGUS NERVE** collection it's composed of **six books** and you'll discover how the vagus nerve is mostly involved in the parasympathetic function of the heart, the lungs, and the digestive system.

Everything you need to get one of them, it's connected to the site you find below.

In add you can join my **Private-Facebook Group** "VAGUS NERVE – KNOW" where you will find many exclusive contents.

WRITE THE URL www.vagusnerve-knox.com/leadbook/

to DOWNLOAD YOUR FREE BOOK
and JOIN OUR EXCLUSIVE COMMUNITY

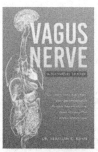 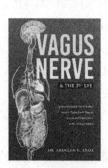 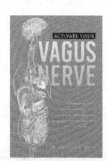
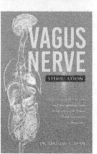 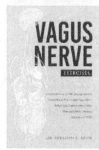 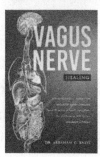

CONTENTS

INTRODUCTION

The vagus nerve's origin is traced in the medulla oblongata of the brain stem, and it falls all the way down to the part of the colon. There are two vagus nerves, twin nerves if you prefer since all the nerves exist in pairs. One emerges from the right side of the medulla oblongata, and the other emerges from the left side; the health experts call them 'the left vagus nerve' and 'the right vagus nerve.' The vagus nerve carries bi-directional traffic, it transmits information from the body organs to the brain and from the brain to the organs back again, thus, creating the gut-brain axis. Several nuclei in the medulla oblongata are associated with the vagus nerve and the different types of information it carries. Those types are mentioned below:

1) The information about the touch, pain and the temperature travels down to the spinal trigeminal nucleus.

2) The sensory information from the internal organs or the visceral sensory information travels to the solitary nucleus.

3) The motor signals originate in the nucleus ambiguous and also the parasympathetic fibers that travel all the way to the heart.

4) The parasympathetic fibers emerge in the dorsal vagal motor nucleus.

The vagus nerve is responsible for the regulation of many critical aspects of human physiology, including heart rate, sweating, blood pressure, speaking, and digestion. This ubiquitous nerve plays a crucial part in controlling the muscles of the throat, the muscles of the voice box, and the immune system. The sources say that according to the latest research, this crucial nerve could be the missing piece of the puzzle, which could enable the treatment of chronic inflammation. It also could let wellness experts discover a cure for various incurable diseases. Sounds fantastic, right? Well, the vagus nerve is a life savior, and it also has more capabilities. You can learn how to unlock them in the chapters below.

CHAPTER 1

The Vagus Nerve and Decision-Making

Some of the world's most successful people decided to skip one decision that people usually pay the most attention to - dressing. Take a look at Obama and Mark Zuckerberg. You'll see that they removed dressing out of their daily lives. They also have made sure to always have the same outfit in their wardrobe in multiple copies.

Decision making is stressful. That is because it is usually done under a constraint of time or more or less critical consequences. The evaluation of the ability to make decisions under these conditions has become a selection criterion in the business world. However, it is known that stress harms most cognitive functions and emotions, even several hours after it happened. As a consequence, it will cause difficulties in getting away from work and being able to rest.

The Connection Between Vagus Nerve And Decision-Making

The vagus nerve is the tenth cranial nerve, and it is the main nerve branch of the parasympathetic system. This system is known to be involved in the modulation of stress. What interests us here is that the Vagus nerve is related to the areas of the brain involved in decision making and the regulation of emotions.

The activity of the vagus nerve can be correlated with a physiological parameter HRV for heart rate variation. HRV is the measure of the variation between heartbeats. This measure has been associated with the vegetative activity of the nervous system. Indirectly, this is how one can know the vagus nerve's behavior. Interestingly, HRV is also positively correlated with brain activity in the region related to decision making in the prefrontal cortex. Therefore, this correlation may indicate that the vagus nerve influences decision making.

Activation of the vagus nerve and its influence on decision-making

The vagus nerve can be activated in various ways - direct or indirect. Directly by electrical stimulation, indirectly by breathing. This activation influences cognitive abilities. For example, artificial stimulation of the vagus nerve improves the photographic memory as well as the time to decide. Similarly, risk aversion and attention control vary with vagal nerve activity (as measured by HRV monitoring). All this indicates the importance of the autonomic nervous system in the use of cognitive functions and, therefore, decision-making.

Vagus nerve activation protects against burnout.

The vagus nerve does not only affect cognitive abilities directly. We have seen above that stress negatively affects decisions. High activity of the vagus nerve results in better recovery from stress after a long day at work. Thus, it has been shown that there is a correlation between the high activity of the vagus nerve and the decreased risk of burnout.

Besides, strong vagal activity leads to better synchronization between the brain, the peripheral immune system, and hormonal reactions to stress. The body avoids being permanently inflamed and overdosed in cortisol that keeps us alert all the time.

It has been so correlated that people with high HRV, or high vagus nerve activity, are healthier, less prone to chronic diseases often related to inflammation, and have a lower risk of cardiovascular problems. A 2013 study shows an inverse correlation between cancer occurrence and vagus nerve activity.

Vagus Nerve's Activity – Breathing And Controlling

The control of the vagus nerve can be done by electrical stimulation. The problem is that it requires surgery. The surgery is not particularly pleasant. Despite that, other ways have been discovered. In other words, breathing. To elaborate, deep breathing methods combined with biofeedback. A biofeedback device has shown to be able to increase the HRV. The mechanism would be three-fold: action on baroreceptors and thus reinforcement of the ability to maintain homeostasis, action on the prefrontal cortex, and direct action on HRV.

Evaluated Respiratory Patterns

Two respiratory reasons were compared to a third control group that breathed without instructions. The respiratory pattern was held for 5 minutes.

The first motif is a motif advocating respiratory symmetry:

✔A count of 5 on inspiration

✔Apnea full of 2 accounts

✔A count of 5 on the expiration

The second pattern imbalances in favor of expiration

✔A 5 count for inspiration

✔Apnea full of 2

✔A 7 count for expiration

In your opinion, what is the most effective reason, and why? The researchers speculated that pattern two would be more effective since expiration stimulates the vagus nerve.

Results Of The Study On HRV And Decision-Making

Two respiratory reasons increase the level of HRV. These patterns can stimulate the vagal nerve. On the other hand, there is no difference between the two in terms of activation level. However, stronger effects were measured with elongated expiration. That is the reason why this one has been used for the measurement of decision-making under stress.

In terms of decision-making, the group with respiratory reasons had statistically much higher results than the group under control stress (more than 50% of success). Equally impressive, the breathing group did not experience increased stress levels, while the control group showed a solid increase in stress markers.

CHAPTER 2

Practical Self Help Exercises for

Activating the Vagus Nerve

Now that you know how the vagus nerve operates and why it is essential for your health let us help you focus on its application. Many people are quick to use any means of vagus nerve activation that comes their way. As already mentioned, there are some techniques of vagus nerve activation that are helpful while others are harmful. You must be cautious not to use dangerous techniques. Continuous activation of the vagus nerve using the wrong techniques may lead to chronic inflammation, which may bring more trouble.

Breathing Techniques for Vagus Nerve Activation

Diaphragmatic breathing can activate the vagus nerve. This type of breathing is capable of reducing the tension on the lungs and the heart. When you use this type of breathing, you allow yourself to breathe in slow bits that help relieve pressure. Diaphragmatic breathing helps in expanding the diaphragm. This is effective because it can reduce blood pressure and, at the same time, can calm down the nerves during anxious moments. The reduction of pressure and calming of nerves helps the body activate parasympathetic actions of the vagus nerve. The activation of parasympathetic activity leads to rest. Here is a step by step guide to diaphragmatic breathing.

Step 1: Position Yourself

When you want to breathe and calm down your nerves, you must align your body to allow sufficient air intake. In simple terms, your lungs should be open. If you try diaphragmatic breathing while lying on your belly or sitting in a wrong position, you will strain; your body should be free enough to allow enough air into your lungs. When you are standing upright or when you are seated upright are the best positions. You can stand in an upright position and slightly spread your arms. This posture opens up your chest to allow sufficient air in. If you are seated on a chair or a mat, ensure that your back is in an upright position. This allows you to inhale the air freely.

Step 2: Inhale and Pause

After positioning yourself, inhale a large chunk of air slowly and hold it in. You can hold your breath for about ten seconds or even more. Given that regular breathing includes 10 - 14 inhalations per minute, the diaphragmatic breathing usually involves around six inhalations per minute. When you inhale the fresh air, do not be in a hurry to let it out. Hold on to it for a few seconds; approximately 10, then release it gently.

Step 3: Slowly Exhale

After about ten seconds, exhale, and start the process all over. When you let out the air, you feel as if space has been freed up, and a weight has been lifted off your shoulders. The exhalation process helps clean your body of all negative energy. When you release the air, you allow your body to calm down and resume normal activities. It is important to note that this type of breathing should be well coordinated to work. If you do not allow yourself to calm down and try focusing on your breath, the effort may be worthless. As much as you want to enjoy your life and get rid of anxiety, you must try training your thoughts to focus on your breathing. It would help if you allowed yourself to visualize the entire process.

Exercises That Activate Your Vagus Nerve

Exercising on a daily basis can also affect your vagus nerve. We know that physical activities are influential and have a positive effect on your heart rate and blood pressure. These activities may moderate the heart rate or may increase it depending on your condition. While physical exercises are effective in controlling the vagus nerve, not all activities will work out. In most cases, it is the gentle physical activities that do not require a lot of energy that works well in activating the vagus nerve. The two main physical exercises used in vagus nerve activation include yoga and tai-chi.

Yoga:

Yoga is a form of physical activity that involves stretching of the body muscles in combination with meditation and affirmation recitations. Yoga is a combination of many physiotherapeutic techniques in one session. You need to find the right yoga trainer if you want to activate your vagus nerve through this type of exercise. The results afterward are quite beneficial. You can also perform yoga at home by using guided videos. One important factor to keep in mind when it comes to performing yoga is that the session should be mind calming. When performing yoga for vagus activation, try incorporating other techniques such as slow breathing, and meditation. To perform yoga well, you will need a quiet location with minimal disruptions. You will also need a yoga mat and a guide video. If you prefer performing among other individuals, you can get into a yoga studio around your home.

Tai-chi:

Tai-chi is a form of wrestling technique originating from ancient China. The course today is performed as a form of exercise. Tai-chi mainly involves slow horizontal movements with the hands placed in front of the practitioner. This type of exercise is calming and very helpful to individuals who wish to stimulate their vagus nerve. If you want to stimulate your vagus nerve, focus on working out on the slow movements. You can use a guided video to perform tai-chi, or you may choose to visit a studio near you.

Aerobic Exercise:

Aerobic exercise is known as the one where you exercise with oxygen. Funny, right? Well, it is not funny at all. After all, it is essential to perform aerobic exercise for vagus nerve stimulation because it helps with heart diseases and blood pressure problems. Now, the question arises, how to perform the aerobic exercise? The answer is simple; it involves:

- Swimming

- Walking

- Running

- Cycling

- Aqua aerobics

- Boxing

These are the activities everyone is familiar with and are super easy to do.

It's that easy, see? All you have to do is swim and walk and ride a bicycle to stimulate your vagus nerve.

Rowing:

The rowing workout is an indoor exercise that involves a machine known as the rowing machine. One can easily workout on it by following the steps mentioned below:

Sit on the machine with a straight back.

Put your feet in the straps and keep yourself straight for a while.

There's an elastic string attached to it which you need to pull to your chest, but your back should be straight as you do so.

Keep pulling the string while bending your knees and leave it slowly, gliding back to the starting position.

Keep repeating it as many times as instructed and then finally let go.

You can increase your time using it and have your vagus nerve stimulated.

Squats:

Squats are one of the easiest exercises for some people. This is the most common exercise that you can easily perform and have your vagus nerve stimulated. Also, by doing squats, you can burn your calories exponentially. Well, do you want to know how to do squats? Follow the steps below:

Begin with standing erect and having your feet wide apart. Your hands should be by your sides.

Now, slowly lift your hands and join them below your chin. Then, slowly push your hips back and fold your knees as if to sit on a chair. Your chest and chin should be up.

Next, rise slowly as if you are standing up from a chair.

Now repeat it 20 times or as instructed.

Easy peasy, lemon squeezy, no?

50 seconds facelift:

A facelift involves the jaw movement, and that is linked with the vagus nerve. When you do this exercise, you cause your vagus nerve to be stimulated instantly. Now, the steps. Well, it's very easy as the name says it all.

Lift your face to the point where you see the front wall meeting the ceiling and close your eyes.

Stay in that position for 50 seconds.

Eventually, release your face and repeat it for 2 to 3 times more.

Sit-ups

Sit-ups are famous, common, and also useful. Some people do these to stimulate their vagus nerve because it has proved to be very helpful in keeping them healthy.

You can do sit-ups by following these steps:

Lay down with your hands under your head and knees bent with feet on the floor.

Now, without straining your neck, sit up slowly and let your thighs touch your torso.

Repeat as instructed.

That was a piece of cake.

Gentle Inversions:

People often go for easy inversion poses that are beneficiary, and Viparita Karani happens to be one of them. It is also known as a leg-up-the-wall pose, and it helps benefit the person by regulating the blood pressure and activating the vagus nerve. The steps involve:

To start it by standing near a wall, make sure you are facing it. Now, keep your toes in contact with the wall where it ends.

Now breathe in and sit on the floor while keeping your toes touching the wall with your knees curved and now extinguish the air from your lungs before keeping your palms on the floor.

Breathe in again and lie down on the floor slowly. Now, breathe out.

Next, put your legs up the wall and keep your hands on the floor on your sides.

Now keep breathing in and out for a few minutes with your eyes closed.

Slowly retreat your legs from the wall and stand back up when you are done.

There you go!

Neck Gnar or Supra-Clavicle Release:

Neck gnar is an exercise where you can ease your neck muscles and have your vagus nerve stimulated. Let's see how you do that:

Seek a wall, take a ball. Yep, it's that easy.

Now, place the ball on your shoulder, right above your clavicle (where your neck meets your shoulder) and sandwich it between you shoulder and the wall.

And, you are done.

3-D Breath breakdown:

This breathing exercise is a must if you want to stimulate your vagus nerve immediately. It's like zen practice. Let's learn how to do that:

Find out a peaceful spot and sit-down crossed leg there.

Now, join your hands as if in a prayer and close your eye.

Next, slow down and breathe in and out while keeping your focus on your breathing.

Keep repeating it until you can focus no more.

And, you're good to go!

Meditation for Vagus Nerve Activation

Meditation is one of the most essential ways of activating the vagus nerve. Any person can use meditation. Even for those that have not attended meditation classes. As compared to tai-chi and yoga, which seem to be complex, meditation is a simple approach.

Meditation involves visualization. The practitioner has to visualize a specific environment that promotes calmness. The main aim of meditation in this process is to calm down the sympathetic action and activate the parasympathetic activity of the vagus nerve. If you are capable of sending a signal to the brain that will initiate the actions of the parasympathetic nervous system, you will be in the right position to move on with your life.

To benefit from meditation, you need to choose the right type of meditation. There are many types of meditation. However, only a few are effective in calming down nerves and boosting your vagus nerve action.

Some of the meditation techniques used to activate the vagus nerve include:

Mindfulness Meditation:

In this type of meditation, the aim is to distract the mind from the thoughts that cause anxiety. When you practice mindfulness meditation, the focus is on yourself. You only think about yourself, your body, your environment. You need to observe the rules for mindful meditation if you want to enjoy the fruits of mindful meditation. First, during mindfulness, a person may discover some frustrating facts about themselves. In mindful meditation, you allow yourself to visualize yourself in a way that you have never done before. Therefore, all the benefits of the meditation should be protected by following the rules.

One of the most important rules of this type of meditation is being non-judgmental. In other words, you are not allowed to judge yourself after observing your thoughts or feelings.

You are required to embrace the truth about yourself. This action promotes calming of nerves.

Some people who suffer from depression only experience nervousness due to fear of being judged. However, if you can learn to accept your flaws through mindfulness meditation, you will not be shaken by anything. Mindfulness meditation teaches you to stand firm and believe in yourself no matter what the world may say about you.

This is the attitude you need to overcome anxiety and depression. This attitude also promotes the parasympathetic activities of the vagus nerve.

Focused Meditation:

Focused meditation is a type of meditation where the practitioner focuses their thoughts on a single object. In this type of meditation, you can choose any item in a room and simply concentrate on it. Focused meditation needs intense concentration.

For instance, you can choose to focus on a chair or a wall. When performing focused meditation, you can't release your eyes from that piece of furniture. Use your mind to describe the chair and try looking at it based on different aspects. Think about its design, colors, shape, make, or any other part of it. Think about factors that make it unique, how it holds weight, among others. This type of meditation is only intended to help you reduce the tension in your mind. After reducing the tension on your mind, the body can slowly lessen the sympathetic actions leading to anxiety.

Peace, Love, and Kindness Meditation:

This is an ideal type of meditation for individuals looking to activate the vagus nerve. The fact that a person may be experiencing anxiety or depression means that they need an activity that will calm down nerves. There is no better activity than peace, love, and kindness meditation.

In this type of meditation, you have to visualize yourself as a center of peace, love, and kindness to the world. In your mind, you have to imagine a world without violence or hate. In this world, you are the primary source of peace, love, and kindness. In this type of meditation, you visualize yourself extending kindness to people who need it.

You stand out as an individual who embraces those who are weak. In your routines, you provide peace and kindness to people who are close to you and show them that the world can be a better place. You freely gift people who need help on the streets. You may also visit your enemies and extend a hand of forgiveness. Create a perfect world in your visualization and indulge in that peaceful world for a few minutes. When you are done with your meditation, you will be in the right place to let go of all your fears and anxiety. This calming effect activates the vagus nerve, allowing you to live an everyday life again.

Transcendental Meditation

Transcendental meditation is a type of spiritual meditation that is mostly spiritually based and focusses on bring an individual's awareness past their physical being or state. It involves the repetition of particular mantras and the use of specific postures to enhance the feeling of inner peace and calmness. Transcendental meditation differs from mindful meditation. Mindful meditation is geared towards bringing attention to the present, and transcendental meditation aims to transcend.

In transcendental meditation, you use the repetition of a mantra to settle your mind and remove all thoughts. It does not involve concentration or focusing on a particular object. Transcendental meditation is typically learned from certified teachers because it requires a precise technique to achieve a transcendental state.

The ultimate result of consistent transcendental meditation is an increased awareness of our existence as part of a large cosmos. It thus helps in shifting thoughts from our person to our surroundings and those around us. It is useful in stress and anxiety reduction and creates a high level of cognitive and thought clarity.

Body Scan Meditation

Stress manifests itself in our bodies as tense muscles, shallow breathing, irregular heartbeat, and overall physical discomfort. It is hard to be aware of how we are feeling each time and what is triggering us to feel a certain way.

Body scan meditation primarily involves examining or scanning your body for areas of tension. The aim is to identify areas where your muscles are tensed or where you have tension knots and essentially relax them to release the tension. The general technique in body scan meditation involves scanning your body from one end to another; for instance, you can start from toe to head. The following steps can help you in practicing body scan meditation;

•   Sit comfortably and relax

•   Slow your breathing drown and focus on deep breathing, which is breathing from your stomach, not your chest.

•   To help you breathe from the belly, you can create a mental image of a balloon inflating and deflating in your stomach as you breathe in and out.

•   Focus on each part of your body and feel for signs of tension, start from your head, and work yourself down systematically through the neck chest abdomen and limbs.

•   During this systematic scanning process, keep doing your deep breathing as it will heighten your awareness and ability to detect tension in your muscles.

•   Notice the general feeling and sensations in different parts of your body, for instance, if you have soreness, tightness, or tense muscles in some part of your body.

•   Once you come across areas on the body that are tense or uncomfortable, focus on those areas as you breathe in and out. You can accompany this focus by gently massaging the area of tension and concentrate on feeling the tension leave your body as you exhale.

•   Do this throughout your body, paying particular attention to the tense and sore areas until you start feeling relaxed in those areas.

Body scan meditation is essential in increasing your body awareness and recognizing when things are going wrong or not working as they should. This type of meditation is a tool that you can use when you are feeling stressed or anxious, and it will help you in releasing tension and becoming more relaxed.

Like in the other types of meditation, our vagus nerve functions best when we are in a relaxed state, so any kind of meditation that helps you relax and get into a peaceful state of mind will be instrumental in activating and stimulating your vagus nerve.

Kundalini Meditation

Kundalini meditation is practiced as part of a type of yoga focused on releasing the energy present at the base of the spine. This energy is referred to as kundalini energy. In Kundalini meditation, the chief goal is to unleash this power at the bottom of the spine and using its energy to cleanse your body of ailments, mental and emotional disorders, and essentially purify your system.

For this type of meditation;

• Increase your awareness and prepare your mind to receive the kundalini energy

• Dress in loose, comfortable clothing and find a quiet, comfortable place for your meditation.

• Cover your head using a shawl or scarf

• Sit with your legs folded and ensure that your spine head and neck are aligned but relaxed

• Close your eyes.

• Practice deep breathing and focus on the inhale and exhale process

• Break down your inhaling with gaps, i.e., breathe in, hold, continue breathing in, hold, and continue. Inhale this way with four pauses and do not exhale during this step

• Once you have done the above process, you can exhale using the same technique, exhale-hold, and continue exhaling. Again, do these four times.

• Do this staggered inhale and exhale process for about four minutes.

• At the end of the four minutes, inhale deeply, bringing your palms together, and holding them together for approximately ten seconds.

• Then exhale deeply and feel your body relax as you exhale.

• As you continue increasing your breathing rate and feeling the breath in your body, you will gradually be able to control your rate and flow of breath. As you go deeper and deeper into these breathing techniques, you should start to uncover the energy at the base of your spine.

The Wim Hof Method

The vagus nerve is connected to many parts of our bodies, and as such, it has been found that we can activate it naturally using these parts of our bodies to stimulate it. An active Vagus nerve means that our bodies can achieve a state of equilibrium between the parasympathetic and sympathetic nervous systems. When either system is not balanced out by the actions of the other, we tend to develop physical and psychological disorders that impact our quality of life.

The Wim Hof method of stimulating the vagus nerve is chiefly based on three main principles, i.e.;

• Cold Exposure

• Breathing

• Commitment

Cold Therapy

Cold therapy, also known as cryotherapy, is one of the pillars of the Wim hof method. Have you ever wondered why a cold compress applied to a bruise or swelling helps reduce pain and speeds up healing? Applying a cold compress reduces blood flow to a particular area, regulates nerve activity, and results in a reduction of inflammation and swelling.

In the same way, cold exposure has multiple health benefits to the body. It has been found to increase weight loss through fat loss, reduce inflammation, and stimulate the secretion and release of feel-good hormones or endorphins in the body. There are several ways you can expose your body to cold therapy. These include;

• Cold showers- these are an easy way to get cold therapy. You can start by turning the water to cold when taking your normal shower. As you build up your cold resistance, you can then go for entirely cold showers. Not only is a cold show invigorating, but it will also get your vagus nerve activated and energize your mind.

•   Ice baths – once you get accustomed to cold showers, you can then graduate to ice baths. The rule of thumb here is not to subject your body to extremes without first building up your stamina. Start with cold showers, and once your body adjusts and can cope with that level of cold exposure, you can gradually move on to ice baths.

Take approximately three bags of ice, put these in a half-full tub. And wait until most of the ice is melted, and the temperature of the bathwater is approximately 59 F degrees.

You can start with limited exposure from 5 to 10 minutes then build up your exposure as your body gets accustomed to the ice water baths. If you notice your body is getting uncomfortable or is in distress at any point during bath, get out as you do not want to harm your body.

After the bath, a hot beverage such as hot cocoa will help you to warm up. You can also go for a short walk to stimulate blood flow. It is important to remember that cold exposure is sensible and that people with pre-existing conditions should not attempt this therapy to avoid causing complications.

Simple Step by Step Guide to Meditation

Step1: Prepare the Meditation Room and Tools

To make meditation successful, you must find a quiet location without interruptions. You can meditate in your bedroom or open space. It is essential that the meditation location has plenty of fresh air and that it allows you to enjoy peace during meditation. You will also need a meditation mat or a right-back chair. You may need some meditation music, but it is not mandatory.

Step 2: Position Yourself for Meditation

Before you start your meditation, ensure that you have enough time to complete the session. Switch off all interruptions such as your cell phone and only use your watch to set a reminder for timing purposes. Position yourself on the mat in a sitting posture with your legs right in front. Sit in an upright position and allow yourself to breathe in the fresh air freely. If you are using a chair, ensure your back is aligned parallel to the straight end of the chair. This allows your back to be in an upright position, which is perfect for free breathing.

Step 3: Close Your Eyes and Focus on Your Breath

To prepare your mind for meditation, you need to draw your concentration. The easiest way to start concentrating is by focusing on your breathing for about 5 minutes. Do not try controlling how you breathe. Just focus your thoughts on it and feel how the air goes in and comes out. This will raise your awareness of the environment and will allow you to concentrate on the moment.

Step 4: Get into Visualization

Once your mind has been prepared for the process, get deep into visualization. With any meditation, you can follow this process. You only start by preparing your room, position yourself, and prepare your mind. Once you are ready, you can now focus your mind on whatever the meditation technique requires. For instance, in focused meditation, you may now open your eyes and choose to focus on the ceiling in the room.

If you know that you will be performing focused meditation, ensure that there is something you can focus on in the room. Interestingly, you cannot lack something to look at and try to describe in your understanding. If you are performing peace, love, and kindness meditation, close your eyes and create the images in your head. You have to start visualizing your activities as the ambassador for peace to those who need it. It is much simple if you close your eyes and only focus on meditation for a given time.

CHAPTER 3

The Vagus Nerve And Glossopharyngeal Nerve (Cranial Nerves IX And X) And Their Disorders

The preganglionic filaments go to the otic ganglion through the lesser shallow petrosal nerve. What's more, postganglionic strands go through the auriculotemporal part of the fifth nerve to reach to arrive at the Parotid organ. The cores of the tactile filaments of the glossopharyngeal nerve are arranged in the petrous ganglion, which exists in the petrous bone beneath the jugular foramen and the unrivaled ganglion, which is little. The exteroceptive filaments supply the faucial tonsils, back mass of the pharynx, some portion of the delicate sense of taste, and taste sensations from the back third of the tongue.

The vagus: This is the longest among all the cranial nerves. The engine filaments emerge from the core ambiguity and supply every one of the pharynx's muscles, with a delicate sense of taste and larynx, except for tensor veli palatine and stylopharyngeus. The parasympathetic filaments emerge from the dorsal efferent core and leave the medulla as preganglionic strands of the craniosacral segment of the autonomic sensory system. They are parasympathetic at work. In this way, vagal incitement produces bradycardia, bronchial tightening, discharge of gastric and pancreatic squeeze, and expanded peristalsis. The tangible part of the vagus has its cores in the jugular in ganglion and ganglion nodosum. The vagus conveys sensations from the back of the outer sound-related meatus and neighboring pinna and torment sensation from the durometer covering the back cranial fossa.

The muffle reflex or the pharyngeal reflex is evoked by applying an improvement, for example, a tongue balde or cotton to the posterior pharyngeal divider or tonsillar locale. When the reflex is available, there will be height and withdrawal of the pharyngeal musculature joined by the tongue's withdrawal. The glossopharyngeal subserves the afferent curve of this reflex while the efferent is through the vagus. This reflex is lost in either ninth or tenth nerve injuries.

Clutters of ninth and tenth nerve capacities

Segregated association of either nerve is uncommon, and as a rule, they are included together, regularly the eleventh and twelfth nerves may likewise be influenced. Glossopharyngeal neuralgia looks like trigeminal neuralgia, yet it is substantially less normal. It happens as severe paroxysmal agony beginning in the throat from the tonsillar fossa. It might be related to bradycardia, and in such cases, it is called vegoglossopharyngeal neuralgia. A preliminary of phenytoin or carbamazepine usually is viable in easing torment. Mind stem injuries like engine neuron ailment, vascular sores, for example, parallel medullary localized necrosis or bulbar poliomyelitis, can influence these nerves together, bringing about bulbar paralysis. Back fossa tumors and basal meningitis may include these nerves outside the cerebrum stem. Complete two-sided vagal loss of motion is incongruent with life. Contribution of the repetitive laryngeal nerves, particularly the left, happens in thoracic sores, and this produces just raspiness of voice without dysphagia.

Turning Your Vagus On

What do nervousness, fractiousness, acid reflux, and restlessness share?

Well, the answer to this question is - pressure. In fact, they are all an outcome from an absence of Vagus action. Your Vagus nerve is significant for your wellbeing and prosperity.

In this book, you'll realize why your Vagus nerve is so essential and how to actuate it to soothe your nerves, rest, condensate better, and bolster your body's characteristic mending powers.

Your Vagus nerve interfaces your cerebrum with your heart, gut, and all your inward organs. Its impact is unavoidable to the point that it has been designated "the skipper" of your parasympathetic sensory system, which is your body's characteristic unwind, remake, and fix reaction group.

Appropriate manipulation of your Vagus nerve holds incessant irritation under tight restraints, putting the brakes on every significant sickness. It directs your heart-beat, amplifying pulse inconstancy, which is a significant marker for heart wellbeing. Furthermore, it flags your lungs to inhale profoundly, taking in the oxygen that renews your imperative vitality.

Your Vagus nerve additionally deciphers fundamental data from your gut to your cerebrum, giving you gut impulses about what is useful or destructive for you. It encourages you to combine recollections, so you recall essential data just as your well-meaning goals.

At last, your Vagus nerve discharges acetylcholine, which counters the adrenaline and cortisol of your pressure reaction, and enacts your body's typical Relaxation Response, with the goal that you can unwind, rest, and let go.

Thus, presently you have an image of why actuating your Vagus nerve is so necessary.

The issue is that our present culture urges us to be so hyper-occupied, so hyper-invigorated, that we keep running in pressure mode always, without knowing it. We are so used to incitement, that we don't have the foggiest idea what genuine unwinding feels like, considerably less how to do it.

Rather than rehearsing a characteristic beat among action and rest, we are hyper-dynamic. What's more, we are so molded that we feel regretful if we're not continually accomplishing something or exhausted in case we're not animated and engaged!

Therefore, nervousness, peevishness, and restlessness are steady mates. This keeps us from resting profoundly and sets us on the way for ceaseless ailments, for example, malignant growth.

Things being what they are, how might we break this risky example?

Luckily, your body is profoundly strong. It is merely hanging tight for you to enact your normal parity, which is as close as a couple of moderate, full breaths away.

At the point when you inhale gradually and profoundly, your Vagus nerve is enacted. It sends quieting signals that moderate your brainwaves and pulse and set moving all the rest and fix systems of your body's regular Relaxation Response.

Along these lines, slow profound breathing is imperatively significant. Be that as it may, there's an issue. Living in steady pressure mode advances an example of limited, fast, shallow relaxation.

In this way, slow profound breathing may take a little practice. Here's a great method to do that:

A Simple Deep Breathing Meditation:

Lie on your back and gently close your eyes. Rest your hands, one over the other, on your lower stomach area.

As you breathe in, enable your lower guts to delicately ascend, as though it is topping off with your breath. As you breathe out, enable your lower mid-region to unwind downwards, as though it is purging out.

Sink into a decent simple cadence, daintily following your breath, as your guts tenderly ascents and falls. Check whether it's conceivable not to constrain this to occur, yet to focus as it usually happens, effectively, easily merely.

As you proceed, check whether you can see the minute you start to breathe in and tail it right until you usually stop. At that point, see the minute you begin to breathe out and follow it right until you typically stop.

Appreciate this calming beat for in any event a couple of minutes- and afterward see how great you feel.

And when you can, feel free to try this out the present moment, so you experience it for yourself...

You can rehearse this straightforward profound breathing reflection once per day to discharge the pressure of the day, and the layers of strain gathered from an earlier time. You can do it lying in bed around evening time before rest, to set up your body to rest profoundly.

In a matter of moments by any means, you'll have reset your body's regular parity, and this will convert into living an increasingly adjusted, glad, and quiet life.

CHAPTER 4

The Human Nervous System

The nervous system is an intricate body of nerves and cells that allows the brain and body to communicate. You could look at it as a large circuit board with channels spanning through the entire body. If this channel or body part is compromised, it affects the body and the brain.

The nervous system is essentially subdivided into two structural areas: the peripheral nervous system and the central nervous system. The central nervous system consists of the spinal cord, nerves, and brain. On the other hand, the peripheral nervous system holds carefully designed cells that are joined to one another and the central nervous system.

Regarding functionality, the peripheral nervous system has two categories: voluntary and involuntary responses. The involuntary responses are processes that occur within the body, such as heart rate and blood pressure, and work without us having to will the function on. The involuntary nervous system is divided into the sympathetic, parasympathetic, and enteric nervous systems. As the name says, the voluntary nervous system is responsible for voluntary muscle movement, like waving your hand or shaking your head.

Sympathetic Nervous System

People are instinctively aware of when they are in danger or feel unsafe. The fight-or-flight response is rooted in this nervous system. It makes us active, causing our pupils to dilate and our heart rate to increase. It can also lead to less saliva production and can hamper digestion.

Parasympathetic Nervous System

This nervous system is also referred to as the "rest and digest" system because it causes the body to react in precisely those terms. This part of the nervous system provides us with a sense of calm. It constricts pupils and slows breathing. Heart rates are slowed, and more saliva is produced, encouraging digestion.

Enteric Nervous System

The enteric nervous system (ENS) is the core nervous system that regulates normal gut function. It encompasses blood sugar levels, blood flow, and mucous secretions.

The ENS operates independently from the parasympathetic and sympathetic nervous systems but can ultimately be influenced by them. The ENS is also said to be the second brain. It is further responsible for peristaltic movements, which ease contents through the stomach, intestines, and colon.

Both the sympathetic and parasympathetic nervous systems have contradictory reactions. One system curbs the response, while the other causes a psychological response.

The vagus nerve travels to almost every part of the body. Hence, when we feel stressed or are faced with emotional turmoil, we experience noticeable abdominal responses, such as a loss or increase in appetite or an upset stomach. Gut reactions are not a figment of our imagination; they are considered genuine nervous signals.

Understanding the Gut-Brain Axis

What is the gut-brain axis? You may ask. Well, this refers to the somewhat complicated relationship between your gut and your brain and the development they have with each other. It deals with the messages that the gut releases to the central nervous system. It refers to the sensitive flora found within the gut that affects all the biochemical signals between the nervous system and the entire gastrointestinal region. This communication highway is the gut-brain axis!

Think about how we salivate when we see a cheesy pizza coming out of the oven. Well, that is all down to the gut-brain axis. Another example is when we feel the need to go to the toilet or develop butterflies in the stomach when we get excited.

One of its most important connections is the one that it has with the vagus nerve, as well as the sympathetic, parasympathetic, and enteric nervous systems. The gut flora influences the vagus nerve, and it lets the brain know the current situation within the intestines.

In related studies, there are investigations on whether the gut flora can influence moods and its link on neurological issues. Individuals who struggle with anxiety and depression tend to struggle with stomach-related problems. There is also a connection between neurological disorders, balance in the gut, and sleep.

The gut flora, an integrated and complicated mix of microorganisms that occupy our digestive tract, holds most of the bacteria compared to other parts of the body. This delicate and balanced environment only begins to develop between one and two years old.

Research has also suggested that those who struggle with autism have gut-related issues and are generally diagnosed with this mental disorder at roughly the same age when gut flora stabilizes, meaning the link between the condition and the flora found in the gut.

All these intricate systems can further affect inflammation in the body and our immune systems by managing what gets used by our bodies and what gets tossed out. If the immune system is in overdrive, it can lead to Alzheimer's disease and depression.

The relationship that humans have with their stomachs is interesting. The stomach provides us energy, incorporates vitamins A and K, and manages the stomach and gut acids. When this environment becomes unbalanced, it can cause autoimmune and inflammatory illnesses. When our diet changes, so do the gastrointestinal environment.

The following foods can benefit your gut-brain axis:

• Foods that are high in tryptophan, such as eggs, cheese, and turkey, hold essential amino acids, which make serotonin, a powerful neurotransmitter.

• Foods that are high in polyphenols, such as olives, coffee, green tea, and cocoa, all increase the healthy flora in our stomachs and intestinal tracts.

• Fiber-rich foods, such as nuts and seeds, fruits, and vegetables:

These food items all hold prebiotic fibers, which lower stress hormones.

• Omega-3-fueled fats: These are some of the most essential nutrients you can take or eat to support your brain and its health. They provide mental prowess and lower the risk of contracting disorders related to the brain.

• Fermented foods, such as yogurt and cheese: Are said to change the activity found within our brains and influence the way we inevitably think and feel. Fermented foods are linked to positive mental health as they combat depression and anxiety, which are associated with gut problems.

By changing the various types of bacteria found within our gastrointestinal tract, we can improve our overall brain health.

Neurons

Each region in the brain and spinal cord (CNS) is made up of many, many cells that are called neurons. Neurons transmit electrochemical signals to communicate with other parts of the body.

Normal cells and neurons do not look alike, although they are each made up of similar components. Neurons are made up of the following three parts:

- Cell Body — this is the core of the neuron and where the nucleus of the cell is housed. The nucleus is the control center of any cell.

- Dendrites — these structures look a bit like roots that extend out from the cell body. The dendrites are the structures that receive signals from the axons of other neurons.

- Axon - is a structure that looks like a long tail; it is what conducts the electrical signals to other neurons, glands, and muscles in the body.

The human body contains around 86 billion neurons that form a complex network of communication channels from various parts of the body to the spinal cord and brain, as well as from the spinal cord and brain to the body. Up until the late 1990s, it was believed that neurogenesis - the process of forming new neurons - only occurred in humans from the time of conception up until the age of 3. After three years of age, it was through that neurogenesis stopped or slowed down. However, researchers at Princeton University found that neurogenesis did occur in certain parts of the adult brain.

Neurons do not all look alike, and they can differ in structure, shape, and size, depending on their use. But they are all made up of the same three parts.

There are three main types of neurons found in the nervous system:

- Interneurons are the most common types of neurons and can be found in the spinal cord and the brain. They are the neurons that pass information from one set of neurons in the spinal cord and brain to another set of neurons.

For example:

- You get a paper cut - your sensory neurons send a signal to the interneuron.

- The interneuron sends an alert to your motor neurons, which is why you jerk your hand away.

- The interneuron sends another signal to your brain, and this is why you feel pain.

- Motor neurons are the neurons that communicate commands from the spinal cord and brain to let them send the signals to the necessary muscles and organs.

For example:

- When you swallow, your motor neurons send a message to the interneurons that, in turn, send the necessary signals from the brain and onto the muscles needed to enable you to swallow.

- Sensory neurons — these are the neurons responsible for communicating various sensations to the brain. Sensations such as:

- Hearing

- Sight

- Smell

- Taste

- Touch

Glial Cells

The nervous system also contains cells that support the neurons, and they are called glial cells. They do not actively process information and instead only keep the neurons. There are just as many, if not more glial cells in the brain than there are neurons.

There are five different types of glial cells:

- Astrocyte — star-shaped cells found in the CNS eliminate brain debris or consume bits of dead neurons, carry nutrients to the neurons, and keep the neurons in position. They create a blood-brain barrier and have reparative functions.

- Microglia — found in the CNS — they aid the neuron by digesting parts of the neuron that has died off.

- Oligodendroglia — located in the CNS — they form tube-like structures called myelin sheaths that support and protect nerves in the central nervous system.

- Satellite cells —cells found in the PNS - offer physical support to the neurons found in the peripheral nervous system.

- Schwann cells — cells found in the PNS — are similar in both look and function to oligodendroglia cells. Still, the Schwann cells (myelin) provide support to the nerves in the peripheral nervous system.

CHAPTER 5

Vagus Nerve dysfunction and how to identify it

Vagus nerve dysfunction results in the loss of consciousness for a few seconds. It is due to the overstimulation of the vagus nerve.

Roles and Functions

- In individuals with weariness, nourishment sensitivities, uneasiness, gut issues, mind mist, and depersonalization, vagal nerve brokenness often impacts everything. These individuals have brought down the vagal volume, which means that the nerve has a lower capacity to play out its abilities.

- The primary inquiry is which part of the vagus nerve is failing, and to what degree it is the issue versus different parts of your ability.

- The vagus nerve is a part of the parasympathetic sensory system, alluded to as the rest-and-digestion system. It's by all account not the only nerve in the parasympathetic system, yet it's by a wide margin the most significant one since it has the most expansive impacts.

- The word vagus signifies "wanderer," since it meanders everywhere throughout the body to different significant organs.

- The vagus nerve influences the cerebrum, gut (digestive organs, stomach), heart, liver, pancreas, gallbladder, kidney, ureter, spleen, lungs, regenerative organs (female), neck (pharynx, larynx, and throat), ears, and tongue.

- Vagus is the most significant nerve in your rest-and-overview framework. You may encounter different medical issues – including acid reflux and anorexia – if your vagus nerve isn't functioning admirably.

Breakdown Causes

Your vagus nerve system can be destroyed in 3 primary manners:

- Communication from an organ to the cerebrum.

- Communication inside the cerebrum.

- Communication from the cerebrum to different territories of the body like the heart, liver, and gut.

How It Affects Your Body

Cerebrum

In the cerebrum, the vagus nerve helps disposition and controls uneasiness and gloom.

The vagus nerve is, to a great extent, liable for the mind-body association since it goes to all the significant organs (aside from the adrenal and thyroid).

It's personally attached to how we interface with each other – it connects straightforwardly to nerves that tune our ears to human discourse, facilitate eye to eye connection, and manages enthusiastic articulations. It impacts the arrival of oxytocin, a hormone that is significant in social holding.

Studies have discovered that higher vagal tone is related to unique closeness to other people and increasingly philanthropic conduct.

Mothers can significantly influence the vagus movement of their kids. Newborn children have lower vagus action when their moms are discouraged, furious, or restless during pregnancy.

A few examinations recommended that the vagus nerve is significant for getting in the psychological condition of "stream." It's accepted that the mix of thoughtful (battle or-flight) and vagus enactment makes the right condition for a stream state.

Vagus nerve incitement may expand alertness (by expanding orexin in the prefrontal cortex). It appeared to diminish the measure of daytime rest and fast eye development in epilepsy patients with horrendous mind damage. Furthermore, they advanced the recovery of awareness in torpid rodents after awful cerebrum damage.

Nonetheless, over activating the vagus nerve may cause 'affliction conduct' (weakness, drowsiness, discouragement, uneasiness, hunger misfortune, torment, brought down inspiration, and inability to focus) when actuated by inflammatory markers in an incendiary state (IL-1b).

Ideal vagus nerve action underpins your emotional wellness and directions with the mind-body association. Overstimulation in provocative states can make you feel drained and restless.

Gut

In the gut, it expands stomach acridity, stomach related juice discharge, and gut stream. Since the vagus nerve is significant for developing gut stream (motility), having less vagus actuation will build your IBS hazard, which is a consequence of a slow stream.

Animating the vagus nerve expands the arrival of histamine by stomach cells, which assists discharge with stomach corrosiveness. Along these lines, low stomach corrosiveness is more often than not, but to some extent, a vagus nerve issue. By discharging the natural factor, the vagus nerve is critical to assist you with engrossing nutrient B12.

To a limited extent, satiety and unwinding following a supper are brought about by initiation of the vagus nerve's transmission to the cerebrum in light of nourishment consumption.

The vagus nerve is highly significant in conditions like GERD, because it controls stomach acidity, yet additionally because it controls the throat.

The vagus nerve bolsters processing by animating stomach corrosive discharge and gut stream. It controls the muscles in your gut and maintains a strategic distance issue, for example, IBS.

Liver, Pancreas, and Gallbladder

In the liver and pancreas, it assists control with blooding glucose balance.

In the gallbladder, it helps to discharge bile, which can assist you with disposing of poisons and separate fat.

Heart

In the heart, it controls pulse and circulatory strain—a promising report on the cardiovascular breakdown that is demonstrated by enhancements with vagal nerve incitement.

Vagus movement animates the liver, pancreas, and gallbladder to advance absorption and glucose control. It likewise brings down pulse and diminishes the danger of coronary illness.

Kidney and Bladder

The vagus nerve advances general kidney work. It assists with glucose control and builds bloodstream, which improves blood filtration. Vagus actuation likewise discharges dopamine in the kidneys, which releases sodium, and subsequently, lowers the pulse.

The vagus nerve additionally goes to the bladder. A symptom of its incitement is urinary maintenance, which implies that less vagus incitement can make you pee now and again. In reality, a significant number of my customers whine about continuous pee (likewise because of low vasopressin, low aldosterone, and high cortisol). The vagus nerve bolsters kidney wellbeing and anticipates visit pee by relieving the bladder.

Spleen

In the spleen, it can lessen the irritation. Note that vagus initiation will reduce irritation in all objective organs (by discharging acetylcholine), yet when it actuates in the spleen, the reaction will most likely be increasingly foundational.

Reproductive Organs

It helps to control fruitfulness and climaxes in ladies by associating with the cervix, uterus, and vagina.

Mouth and Ears

In the tongue, it helps control taste and saliva, while in the eyes, it helps to discharge tears.

The vagus nerve clarifies why an individual may hack when tickled on the ear, for example, when attempting to evacuate ear wax with a cotton swab.

Vagus nerve incitement helps individuals with tinnitus in light of its association with the ear.

The vagus nerve invigorates the spleen, conceptive organs, and organs in your ears and mouth.

Potential Symptoms of Low Vagal Tone

- Depression.

- Obesity and weight gain.

- Anxiety.

- Brain problems.

- IBS.

- Chronic fatigue.

- High or low heart rate.

- Difficulty swallowing.

- Gastroparesis, also known as delayed gastric emptying.

- Heartburn.

- Dizziness/fainting.

- B12 deficiency.

- Chronic inflammation.

Conditions That May Improve From Vagus Activation

- Since the vagus nerve is associated with many different functions and brain regions, research distinctively shows the positive effects of vagal stimulation on a variety of conditions, including but not limited to:

- Cancer.

- Anxiety Disorders.

- Autism.

- Heart disease.

- OCD.

- Alzheimer's.

- Migraines.

- Fibromyalgia.

- Obesity.

- Tinnitus.

- Alcohol addiction.

- Bulimia.

- Multiple sclerosis.

- Chronic heart failure.

- Memory disorders.

- Mood disorders.

- Bad blood circulation.

- Leaky Gut.

- Severe mental diseases.

Potential Manifestations of Harm to the Vagus Nerve Include:

- Trouble talking or loss of voice.

- A voice that is dry or wheezy.

- Issue drinking fluids.

- Loss of the muffle reflex.

- Pain in the ear.

- Abnormal pulse.

- Irregular pulse.

- Diminished generation of stomach corrosiveness.

- Sickness or heaving.

- Stomach swelling or pain.

The Side Effects that a Person May Have to Rely upon is When Some Portion of the Nerve is Harmed

Gastroparesis

Specialists accept that harm to the vagus nerve may likewise cause a condition called gastroparesis. This condition influences the stomach related framework's automatic constrictions, which keeps the stomach from appropriately exhausting.

Side effects of gastroparesis include:

- Sickness or regurgitating, particularly heaving undigested nourishment hours after eating.

- Loss of hunger or feeling full not long after beginning a dinner.

- Indigestion.

- Stomach pain or swelling.

- Unexplained weight reduction.

- Vacillations in glucose.

A few people create gastroparesis after experiencing a vagotomy system, which expels all or part of the vagus nerve.

Vasovagal Syncope

At times the vagus nerve overcompensates to certain pressure triggers, for example,

- Introduction to extraordinary warmth.

- Dread of real mischief.

- Seeing blood or having blood drawn.

- Stressing, including attempting to having a solid discharge.

- Staying quite a while.

Keep in mind that the vagus nerve animates specific muscles in the heart that help to slow pulse. At the point when it goes overboard, it can cause an unexpected drop in pulse and circulatory strain, thereby bringing about blacking out. This is known as vasovagal syncope.

Vagus Nerve Testing

To test the vagus nerve, a specialist may check the stifler reflex. During this piece of the assessment, the specialist may utilize a soft cotton swab to tickle the back of the throat on the two sides. This should make the individual stifler. If the individual doesn't choke, this might be because of an issue with the vagus nerve.

CHAPTER 6

Health and Life Benefits

The vagus nerve is responsible for keeping many organs functioning well by keeping the brain-organs connection intact. It wanders from the brainstem through the heart, lungs, stomach, and intestines, only stopping in the colon; thus, it is it deals with all the problems occurring in its region.

Once stimulated, the vagus nerve can help people have a normal heart rate, ideal blood pressure level, no gastrointestinal problem, and many other jaw-dropping benefits.

The Methods which you Can Activate your Vagus Nerve

Battles Epilepsy:

The vagus nerve is a conduit of sensory and motor information between the brain and its associated organs. The crucial information it carries helps stop the brain cells from emitting signals in an uncontrollable fashion, halting the overexcitement of the brain and reducing seizures caused by epilepsy. The vagus nerve stimulation is not only for the treatment of epileptic seizures but also for the seizures caused by an injury or inflammation. The vagus nerve stimulation works even when the anti-seizure drugs abstain from being of any use, and this phenomenon makes the VNS successful and a healthy activity.

Combats Chronic Inflammation:

The vagus nerve is responsible for dealing with the 'rest-and-digest' and the 'tend-and-befriend' reflex. When you stimulate the vagus nerve, it forces the brain to function and order the inflammation reflex to die down at once without using any drugs, and the other organs are forced to listen to what brains say since it is the power hub of the body. This all occurs when the state of inner calmness is achieved, which ultimately tames the inflammation.

According to the research conducted by the experts from Amsterdam and the US together, the vagus nerve stimulation inhibits the pro-inflammatory cytokines, which cause the arthritis inflammation or general inflammation to disappear, which automatically lowers the chances of obesity and cancer pathogenesis since these two are closely linked with the inflammation problem. Also, there is a disease known as Crohn's disease, which refers to the inflammation of the digestive tract, which causes diarrhea, pain in the abdomen, weight loss, fatigue, and other problems. But we have our hero, the vagus nerve to stimulate and put to work! It inhibits this plaguing disease altogether.

Normalizing the Heart Rate:

The vagus nerve stimulation enables the process of normalizing the heart rate quickly. People root for slow and deep belly breathing methods to help better their heart rate. This becomes possible when the sensory and motor fibers present inside the vagus nerve and let it keep track of the heartbeat rhythm and when the brain doesn't find it good enough, it commands the heart rate to either slow down or increases according to the situation. What a fantastic health benefit!

As if that's not enough, the vagus nerve activation also prevents heart failure and other cardiovascular diseases.

Gets Rid of Anxiety and Depression:

This is another health benefit that vagus nerve stimulation offers. The anxiety sticks to people like a second skin, and depression never abandons them as if it is the most loyal thing to ever exist on planet earth, but just doing one task could help you unfriend both this duo in no time. Only activate your vagus nerve through various tips and techniques given in this book and enjoy a peaceful life with no nuisance.

Betters the Blood Pressure:

The most powerful, X cranial nerve in the human body is also in charge of dealing with the blood pressure level of a human body. It not only identifies the variation in it but also improves it if the improvement is needed. This happens when a person undergoes an experience that causes the fear or any negative feeling to surface, which lets the person lose their calm and have their heart rate and blood pressure level either increased or decreased. When electrified, the vagus nerve takes the matter in its hands and, with a little effort, helps the situation come under control.

Turns the Stress off:

The vagus nerve stimulation is responsible for abruptly turning off the stress by taking control of the stress hormone, cortisol. It stops the reaction from occurring which causes the stress to surface.

Helps with Rapid Cycling Bipolar Disorder:

FDA approved vagus nerve stimulation for bipolar disorder in 2005. When the natural or surgical process stimulates the X cranial nerve, it causes the brain to alert itself and carry proper instructions. This could help the patient with rapid cycling bipolar disorder to live a healthy life.

Develop New Brain Cells:

The brain is closely connected with the vagus nerve, which causes it to perform the task of carrying sensory and motor information within the brain well. Hence, when the vagus nerve is activated, it performs better. Resulting in new brain cells that prove to be very beneficiary for the body and other organs since the brain itself is the powerhouse of the body.

Sharpens the Memory:

The vagus nerve stimulation is responsible for improving the memory of a person, which is also linked to cortisol secretion. And when it does so, the person efficiently battles Alzheimer's disease.

Helps Tackle the Problems of Gastrointestinal Tract:

Since the vagus nerve is a part of the parasympathetic nervous system, it deals with the problems occurring in the gastrointestinal tract. The vagus nerve travels through various organs among which the gastrointestinal tract comes; hence when the vagus nerve is stimulated, it helps the person tackle the digestion and excretion problems, it balances the appetite, and it also deals with the hormones causing hunger and feeling of stomach fullness. It is reported even to help drive out the problem caused by diabetes known as gastroparesis; which refers to delayed gastric emptying.

Forces the Lung to Breath:

By the activation of the vagus nerve, the lungs can breathe well. The sensory nodes on the lungs connect the brain with the lungs when the X cranial nerve is stimulated. This causes the lungs to breath when the brain commands it to. This is why people go through any incidents that shake them, and the vagus nerve stimulation causes the lung to keep the breathing steady. It also causes the prevention of lung failure which is like a cherry atop the cake.

Helps Control Pain in Fibromyalgia:

The fibromyalgia disease causes the brain to receive pain signals, whereas the vagus nerve stimulation stops the process and help reduce the pain in no time. You can either use the natural VNS method, or you can get the VNS device implant. Regardless, the results are excellent, and people recommend it all the time.

It Causes you to Bid Farewell to Migraine Headache:

The signals transferring through the vagus nerve help reduce the migraine pain when you activate your X cranial nerve. Isn't that nice to hear? Especially when you or your loved one is suffering from this clingy disease. Just take slow, deep breaths, wash your face with cold water, or adapt any other method to kick-start your vagus nerve into action.

Treats all Kind of Abdominal Pain:

The vagus nerve stimulation is a non-drug therapy for all kinds of abdominal pain since the vagus nerve falls in the abdomen, affecting it simultaneously. The abdominal pains are caused due to inflammation; at times, they occur due to injury and other problems. But, vagus nerve stimulation has this fantastic health benefit. It makes sure that your abdominal pains are defeated, and you are happy and healthy.

It is a Line of Defence Against Obesity:

This unique health benefit is only due to the stimulation of your vagus nerve. The X cranial nerve is responsible for helping people prevent weight gain by causing variation in metabolism and decreasing fat stores. Also, some teens and adults are prone to have a habit of depressing eating; hence, when VNS treats the bone of contention; depression, it ultimately helps people increase the distance between them and obesity. What an easy way!

It prevents Stroke and TB:

When the vagus nerve is electrified, it affects the level of acetylcholine, which causes the neurotransmitter's rebalancing, resulting in the prevention of stroke and tuberculosis. This is one fantastic health benefit that only the stimulation of the X cranial nerve can provide. Amused? Well, sit tight, there are more to come.

It Prevents the Oxidizing Agents from Deteriorating the Brain:

The vagus nerve stimulation forces all the oxidizing agents like cortisol to stop before they reach the brain and deteriorate it. People practice meditation and yoga for this very purpose and end up triggering their vagus nerve to be electrified and help their brain to stay away from deterioration.

It Enables People to Sleep Better:

When people are in rest mode, they cause their vagus nerve to come to life. It takes charge of their heart rate and blood pressure. This causes the body to calm and abandon all the worries out. The sleep soon kicks in once the vagus nerve carries out the brain's command to all the organs which relax as soon as they get the message. Next time you have trouble sleeping, all you have to do is stimulate your X cranial nerve and voila!

Works as a Catalyst in Human Growth Process:

The vagus nerve stimulation is proved to help speed up the process of human growth, didn't know that, did you? Well, now, you know. While the body is at rest, all the organs and the systems let growth become possible. All thanks to the vagus nerve which gets activated and enables you to grow exponentially.

It Rids you of the Insulin Resistance:

X cranial nerve activation indirectly proves to be very useful for diabetic patients. It controls bodily fluids, which are harmful and greatly benefit people as they strive to live a healthy life. The insulin resistance in diabetic patients is widespread, but vagus nerve stimulation comes to the rescue and helps the person get rid of it in just a few deep breaths! Very convenient.

Vagus Nerve Stimulation and the Medical Science:

The success of vagus nerve stimulation has taken people by surprise. It has sky-rocketed over the past few years and managed to secure its feet in medicine. A new field in medicine is reported to birth according to the sources. It is known as bioelectronics, and it includes implant for sending electric impulses to different parts of the body. This field would give solutions and cures of countless problems and diseases without any drug or fewer of them. It would be a non-drug treatment. Wellness experts are rooting for this unique benefit, and you can't question why!

What Causes Vagus Nerve Disorders?

Harm to the vagus nerve can be avoided now and then, while in others, another infirmity or injury might be the reason.

Providing engine nerve driving forces from the tongue and voice box muscles, just as getting tangible motivations from the chest and mid-region organs, ear, and throat, is a difficult task.

Add sending instinctive nerve heartbeats to the stomach and chest organ organs, and throat organs, and there is space for lamentable accidents en route. In that capacity, vagus nerve harm can be brought about by:

<u>Constant Alcohol Abuse</u>

Constant liquor misuse is a lot of nothing for the autonomic sensory system, as it has a poisonous, portion-related impact. Strikingly, the vagus nerve is one of those that can be hurtfully influenced by this kind of misuse.

This maltreatment, known as alcoholic neuropathy, makes harm various nerves. Sadly, if a more significant number of nerves than the vagus are influenced, side effects can be significantly progressively dangerous for the body's general working.

Diabetes

Predictable increment in glucose can prompt changed nerve science. As this infection can bring about nerve harm to a significant number of them, the vagus nerve doesn't get away.

Gastroparesis is one of the primary consequences of diabetes-prompted harm to the nerve. In like manner, side effects incorporate clogging, spewing, and stomach swell.

Fundamentally, the stomach and digestive system muscles are never again ready to move nourishment appropriately around appropriately.

Complexities during Surgeries

During medical procedures concentrated on the small digestive system or stomach, the vagus nerve can be harmed. One that is generally connected with this sort of harm is the laparoscopic Hemi fundoplication. In this manner, this method is utilized as a treatment for gastric reflux.

Diseases

Upper respiratory viral diseases infer another offender as it identifies with vagus nerve harm.

It may be difficult to bind if there has been harm at first, as side effects appear to be a standard cold or gentle influenza. Conceivably, they incorporate nasal clog, runny nose, and hack.

It becomes more apparent that there might be vagus harm when side effects stay long. Subsequently, should vagus nerve harm be the reason; it is spoken to as viral vagal neuropathy or PVVN.

A few people experience the ill effects of issues talking appropriately, such as throat clearing, vocal weariness, and diligent hack.

As we plunge further into the vagus nerve's universe, it tends to be somewhat startling, thinking about the manners in which it tends to be influenced.

Consecutively, the uplifting news that we bring means a few different ways to treat the clutters and turn around the harm.

The Vagus Nerve and Chronic Pancreatitis

Chronic pancreatitis is a part of inflammation diseases, and it is also connected with the gut. The pancreas is situated right behind the stomach and is responsible for producing special protein enzymes that help the food to be digested. Moreover, the pancreas also controls the level of sugar in the blood by secreting certain hormones.

Now, chronic pancreatitis occurs when inflammation occurs in the pancreas. There are two types of pancreatitis: acute, lasting for a few days, usually don't come back, and chronic pancreatitis occurs when the inflammation fails to be eliminated and keeps returning. Also, atop that, it lasts for months and years and keeps growing severe. Chronic pancreatitis causes permanent damage to the pancreas.

The stones of calcium and also the cysts might occur in it too. This would cause blockage to appear in the pancreas, which would prevent the digestive enzymes and fluid from being transferred to the stomach. The stomach would then have trouble digesting food and regulating the level of sugar in the blood and keeping diabetes at bay. Also, it usually occurs in people aging from 30 to 40.

What possibly might be the causes of chronic pancreatitis? Well, they are mentioned below:

- Autoimmune disease

- A narrow pancreatic duct

- A blockage of the pancreatic duct (it carries enzymes from the pancreas to the small intestine).

- Cystic fibrosis is a hereditary problem that involves mucus to be generated in the lungs.

- Hypercalcemia

- Hypertriglyceridemia

Well, other than these, some other factors that are responsible for causing chronic pancreatitis are excessive alcoholism, smoking addiction, and living in the tropical regions of Asia and Africa because there are chances of malnutrition according to some sources.

You need to identify it before dealing with it, and that is possible only when you know the symptoms of chronic pancreatitis. Let's go through these various symptoms it shows:

- Nausea and vomiting

- Fatty, loose stale

- Excessive thirst

- Diarrhea

- Fatigue

- Upper abdominal pain

- Unexplained weight loss

- Shortness of breath

- Pancreatic juice would be found in the abdomen

Some diseases emerge as the symptoms of chronic pancreatitis; those are:

- Intestinal blockage

- Jaundice

- Internal bleeding

The pain also occurs, which makes it unbearable even to breathe, let alone eat or drink.

Now, chronic pancreatitis has been discussed at length, and they are often diagnosed by the following:

- X-rays

- MRI scan

- CT scan

- Ultrasound

There is also one magical cure for chronic pancreatitis that is the vagus nerve stimulation. Now let's discuss the treatment!

The vagus nerve carries the sensory information to the CNS (Central Nervous System). The vagus nerve is a pathway basically where the bi-directional flow of information occurs from the gut to the brain and then from the brain to the gut. Hence, when chronic pancreatitis occurs, it ultimately knows that it has to send signals to the brain regarding the occurrence of chronic pancreatitis. The pain during this condition is unbearable, and the patient has to take a painkiller. But to stop both the disease to strengthen its root and the pain, one of the best cures is the vagus nerve stimulation by:

- Deep, belly breathing.

- Non-invasive transcutaneous vagus nerve stimulation

Now, by using these processes, the pain sensitivity was seen decreasing. And, also, the gut motility was improved by these two methods. This proved that the modulation of the vagal tone index is beneficial in dealing with specific diseases involving gut problems and inflammation. The vagus nerve is a crucial part of the immune system, and when stimulated, it proves to be helpful in multiple diseases.

The Vagus Nerve and Irritable Bowel Syndrome

Irritable bowel syndrome or IBS is a very troublesome disease. It involves altered bowel habits, such as:

- Bloating

- Gas

- Diarrhea

- Chronic constipation

- Severe pain and discomfort in the abdomen

This disease is not necessarily a serious one and is not known as "life-threatening," but the symptoms keep the person troubled and cause unrest to develop in their mind. The bi-direction interaction between the gut and the brain, thus, creating a brain-gut axis, is the one that holds the balance maintained in the gastrointestinal tract.

The leading cause is still not discovered of this disease. But, a few sources say that Irritable Bowel Syndrome is usually caused by specific allergies or stress (either physical or mental). At times, it is reported to be transferred from one of the parents. The changes in one's lifestyle, environment, and other areas are responsible for contributing to the occurrence of IBS. But there is a cure to IBS that would help you get rid of it without much effort. Want to know what that cure is? What are you waiting for then? Let's dive in!

To be sincere, there is not only one but tons of other cures present to deal with the Irritable Bowel Syndrome. But those other cures involve drugs or medicine intake, which have many side-effects etched to them. Therefore, a less problematic and drug-free solution to deal with IBS is the vagus nerve stimulation.

Some people, however, also root for identifying the cause first regarding the vagus nerve. They look for any damage in the vagus nerve and examine it to see if it's the vagus nerve dysfunction that is causing the IBS to occur since it is the pathway between the gut and the brain that deals with all the aspects of the gastrointestinal tract. But if they fail to find any damage, they seek to activate the vagus nerve to maintain the vagal tone index. And that does all the work for them. The vagus nerve communicates with the brain about the problems occurring, and the brain jumps into action to solve all the issues, including bloating, gas, abdominal pain, and other symptoms

IBS brings. The stomach acid runs low during IBS, and the vagus nerve makes sure that this doesn't happen by causing the cells to release histamine, which creates the stomach acid that the body needs to break the food down. Now, when the vagus nerve is activated through multiple safe ways, it provides various other benefits such as:

- Promotes relaxation

- Balances heart rate

- Eradicates anxiety

- Alleviate depression

- Controls blood pressure

And many other countless benefits occur when one keeps the health of the vagus nerve in check and makes sure that it is stimulated safely and effectively eradicating all the troubles that come their way. Well, it doesn't end here; there is more to the vagus nerve that you need to unveil.

Methods for Vagus Nerve Incitement:

Yoga and Meditation - both of these things increment parasympathetic framework movement. Attempt a couple "Oms" the vagus nerve adores it.

- Breathing gradually and profoundly from your stomach

- Exercise-The gut stream is invigorated by mellow exercise.

- Oxytocin

- Positive social associations

- Fasting

- Letting your body conform to cold - cold water in the face, cold showers, and so on

- Acupuncture

- Zinc

- Gargling - gets the muscles at the back of the throat, which helps in incitement.

- Massage

- Probiotics

- Chanting or Singing

- Laughter - can indeed be the best prescription.

- Eating Fiber

- Laying on your correct side when dozing

Likely, the rundown comes as a broad one with the end goal that it controls your day-by-day exercises. It additionally incorporates rehearses like straining stomach muscles or hacking, rehearsing Tai Chi, which expands pulse and getting some sun.

Eventually, the simple things that we do each day appear to have a massive effect on our vagus nerve.

Vagus Nerve And Migraines

The vagus nerve can be used to help eliminate or reduce migraines significantly. The best part is, we all have a vagus nerve and can use it. It is not certainly known whether vagus nerve stimulation can definitely help with migraines because that field is not entirely explored. However, several research studies show that people who received vagus nerve stimulation over multiple years reported a significant improvement in their migraines. This also happened in frequency and pain level.

A survey conducted by Southern Illinois University for individuals who received vagus nerve stimulation for epilepsy showed that multiple people who had migraines before the therapy reported vast improvements in frequency and pain levels. All of the people who did have migraines before the treatments report vast improvements afterward. This is a strong indication that vagus nerve stimulation significantly positively impacts migraines. Of course, these simulations were done medically using implanted devices. However, many of the techniques we discussed can still have minor, indirect effects.

Many other prominent studies have shown that stimulation of the vagus nerve, including the noninvasive approach, significantly reduces migraines for many individuals. This further cements that direct nerve stimulation is not necessary to help relieve migraines. The reporting in the reduction of pain is done by the patients themselves, which is the strongest indication. If a person states they are not in pain, then they are not in pain. Many of these individuals also reported a higher quality of life due to the lack of pain. When a person has less pain, they are more likely to continue healthy practices as well.

A study done by a prominent neurologist in the early 2000s discusses a patient he had with chronic epileptic seizures. Unfortunately, for whatever reason, the Vagus nerve stimulation did not improve epilepsy. Not every therapy will work for every individual as each human organism is unique in its own way. This was an unfortunate circumstance for this patient.

However, they were surprised to learn that the patient had a significant reduction in his chronic migraines. The patient went under treatment for something else and cured something never planned to fix it. That is amazing not only for the patient but also for all the people that seek relief for migraines. This was not the intended result, but since it worked, the treatment was partially successful. Researchers are continuing to do further studies on this phenomenon between the vagus nerve and migraines. It was found by accident as multiple people who were getting treated for seizures using stimulation, surprisingly had an improvement in their migraines and headaches.

The parasympathetic response of the vagus nerve seems to reduce and even eliminate the causes of severe migraines significantly. The parasympathetic response likely inhibits the sympathetic nervous system's overstimulation in these cases, effectively altering the pain response. Vagus nerve stimulation also reduces stress, which can be a trigger for migraines. When the sympathetic nervous system is elevated, stress is increased. When the parasympathetic inhibitory response kicks in, stress, and in turn, pain, is significantly decreased

Next time that migraine hits, try some of the techniques we discussed earlier. Go for a long walk or hit the gym. This may be difficult as exercise will be the last thing on your mind. You can also sit and take some deep breaths, hum, or take a cold shower. Whatever looks right for you at that particular and, at the same time, complicated moment, try it out. Stimulating and utilizing the full potential of the vagus nerve can vastly improve migraines and improve your quality of life.

Vagus Nerve and Depression

Depression, or major depressive disorder, is a mood disorder that causes a person to have persistent feelings of sadness and loss of interest. Depression can affect a person mentally and physically and take a significant toll on a person's daily activities. It is an illness, just like any other, that can cause a person not to want to face life and become secluded. Even though mental health is gaining prominence and becoming accepted by the general population, a significant segment of the population does not take it seriously.

They feel that a person can snap out of it. This is not the case. A person cannot just snap out of it. Depression is more than just getting over something. It is an illness that may require medical attention. There is a difference between having a day off, and a major depressive disorder that significantly reduces your ability to function every day. When a person is suffering from severe depression, they are often walking a thin line, and one little thing could push them over the edge. For this reason, their feelings and mood disorders always need to be validated. They need to be taken seriously.

Untreated depression can lead to extensive pain and trauma. Severe depression may lead to self-harm. There are many tragic stories of people who did not reach out for help, out of fear of appearing weak, and things took a turn for the worse. We do not want this to happen to anybody because they felt like they could not reach out to someone.

Depression is not something to take lightly, and if a person is exhibiting the signs of depression, it must be taken seriously. There are many signs and symptoms of depression that must be considered. Among them are feelings of sadness and tearfulness, anxiety, reduced appetite, unexplained physical problems, feelings of worthlessness, seclusion, loss of interest, anger, frustration, always blaming themselves, and many other things. Take special notice when someone suddenly stops doing something they have always loved to do. Also, give special attention to notable mood swings.

Next time a person you know and love is experiencing symptoms of depression, don't get annoyed. Depression is an illness, just like diabetes, and a person suffering from it needs support, and not be told to get over it. Perhaps using the natural techniques for vagus nerve stimulation may be beneficial for them. Once again, it may not cure their depression, but it will improve their mood and ability to live life tremendously.

If vagus nerve stimulation continues to inhibit depression effectively, then maybe the stigma that still exists around mental illness can be eliminated once and for all. This may be the most outstanding result of all. Even people who have mental illness feel guilty. We don't hear people apologizing for heart disease. But they still apologize for being depressed. This needs to stop, and increased vagus nerve stimulation can help.

Here is one suggestion that will help all parties involved. When helping a friend who is experiencing depression, take them out to have some fun. Remember that laughing and having a good time helps to stimulate the vagus nerve. Take your friend out for a night on the town, and you may help with their depression.

Vagus Nerve and PTSD

Post-Traumatic Stress Disorder, or PTSD, is a mental condition caused by a traumatic event that had a severe impact on someone. The people who are affected most commonly are in the military, law enforcement, first responders, or anyone in a field where tragedy is a common occurrence. However, PTSD may also strike just about anybody and everybody who has been through a traumatic event. A serious accident, death of a loved one, getting assaulted, or any number of tragic events may cause a person to have PTSD.

It may take years to overcome PTSD, and some never overcome it at all. PTSD can manifest itself in multiple ways, including anxiety, anger, nervousness, negative thoughts, flashbacks, and chronic pain. They will often re-experience the trauma various times in their heads. There is a significant split, even within the military community, whether or not PTSD is legitimate.

For this reason, just like with depression, people will dismiss it as a non-issue. They believe that someone can get over it. A person cannot only get over it, though. PTSD is very real and is a severe mental disorder that needs to be treated as such. Unfortunately, PTSD continues to carry a negative stigma to it that can hopefully be a thing of the past once people start realizing some of the physical elements to it as well.

While there is no known cure for PTSD, there are therapies that may be used to help subside some of the signs and symptoms. Currently, some of the treatments include talk therapy and exposure therapy. Several studies suggest that vagus nerve stimulation may be a useful adjunct therapy for helping with PTSD, especially with its associated pain. A University of Texas, Dallas, made a study in which the effects of vagus nerve stimulation on rats were researched. The rats in this particular study displayed some signs that come with PTSD, like fear, aggression, and anxiety.

A session of vagus nerve stimulation showed a significant reduction in these negative signs. Not only that, but the signs also did not return in many cases after another episode of trauma, suggesting that the stimulation may have more long-term effects than the other therapies. Researchers feel that if the stimulation can work in the same manner in humans, it may significantly reduce the pain associated with PTSD. If the effects are more long term as well, then it is undoubtedly an adjunct therapy worth looking into.

If you have a friend or loved one who experiences PTSD, perhaps it is time to work on them. Please help them by using the techniques that will stimulate their vagus nerve. That old cliché of "laughter is the best medicine" may be the ultimate tool. Help your loved one get regular exercise. Remember, this does not just mean going to the gym. Most people are more likely to do something if they enjoy it.

Find something they want to do physically and help them do it. If they love playing basketball, play a quick pickup game. If they love going for walks, find a nice trail, and enjoy the sites. Whatever you can do to get them moving, do it. Finally, how about a nice round of karaoke? Singing and dancing are definitely a great way to stimulate the vagus nerve and get your friends out of the poor mental state they are in.

If we can continue to correlate vagus nerve stimulation with helping to subside the signs of PTSD, we can hopefully remove the stigma associated with it. Just like with depression, we may never be able to cure PTSD, but we can certainly manage it with the appropriate practices.

We want to talk about how PTSD can manifest itself into physical symptoms like muscle tightness, chest pain, fatigue, and digestive issues. Many of these physical responses to a traumatic event indicate a sympathetic nervous system activity. Things like muscle tightness and chest pain that are not heart-related often come from stress and being worked up for so long. They do not come from being in a relaxed state.

Furthermore, fatigue develops when the body is overly stressed for long periods. This is why excessive sympathetic responses are not healthy for the body. If your body is in a constant state of pain and tiredness due to a traumatic event, then perhaps it is time to stimulate your vagus nerve to inactivate your parasympathetic response. The parasympathetic response inhibition will put your body in a state of relaxation, releasing the built-up tension and helping reduce the pain associated with PTSD. Do this regularly, and it can help to manage the negative signs and symptoms of Post-Traumatic Stress Disorder.

Vagus Nerve and Inflammation

Does the vagus nerve help with inflammation? Yes, it does. Inflammation, also known as the inflammatory response, is your body's natural response to a variety of things, such as stress. The inflammatory response occurs under many circumstances, especially when our body is trying to fight off disease. Mild inflammation is needed for the body to maintain its proper functions. When the body perceives a threat like an illness or injury, the inflammatory response kicks in to subdue the threat.

This can be marked by swelling, pain, fevers, and fatigue. Once again, inflammation is needed to help out bodies maintain their functionality. However, excessive or untreated inflammation can create many health problems throughout the body. In cases of stress, inflammation may occur due to the sympathetic nervous system's fight or flight response. In general, whenever the body perceives any threat, it inhibits the parasympathetic nervous system and stimulates the sympathetic reaction so that it can deal with the perceived threat. This is why you will notice an increase in heart rate when a person has an infection. The body is becoming stimulated to defend itself.

Since the vagus nerve is the main component of the parasympathetic nervous system, proper stimulation will help to counteract the sympathetic nervous system, effectively reducing inflammation. Especially in the case of inflammation, which can occur for several reasons, it is of great importance to stimulate the vagus nerve regularly.

While many other interventions may need to be done to combat chronic inflammation, exercises to stimulate and activate the vagus nerve are an appropriate adjunct therapy to help suppress the sympathetic nervous. An excessive, heightened response will eventually have detrimental health consequences. The vagus nerve's ability to control inflammation through the parasympathetic response showcases its ability to affect the immune system indirectly, which produces the inflammatory response mechanism.

Stress is a significant trigger for the inflammatory response also. Indicating even further, the sympathetic nervous system is at play here. In this case, things like deep breathing and humming will effectively reduce stress, inhibit the sympathetic response, stimulate the vagus nerve, and ultimately reduce inflammation. When stimulated to its full potential, the vagus nerve can strongly influence the immune system, thereby affecting good health. The vagus nerve is looking stronger and stronger the more we talk about it.

Vagus Nerve and Fibromyalgia

There is still not much known about fibromyalgia as the pain does not come from a specific cause or area in the body. Many researchers believe that with fibromyalgia, painful sensations are amplified due to the way the brain processes pain. A real reason is not fully known regarding this issue.

Sometimes the pain is triggered by a particular event, like an accident or surgery. Other times, there is no single experience, but the pain just seems to accumulate over time. There is no cure for fibromyalgia at this moment. However, there are interventions, both medical and nonmedical, that can help with subsiding the symptoms that come with it. Once again, our friend, the vagus nerve, is at play here.

In a 2011 NIH study, the leading researchers suggested that vagus nerve stimulation may be a useful adjunct treatment for fibromyalgia patients. Further research was definitely needed, though. Many researchers feel that vagus nerve stimulation is effective in treating pain because it is able to negate a wide variety of factors that contribute to pain, like inflammation and the pain response. There is still much that is up in the air about fibromyalgia. However, the results of studies continue to suggest that the pain associated with it is significantly reduced with vagus nerve stimulation. Pain is often heightened during times when the body is at stress. Since the vagus nerve can lower a person's stress through the sympathetic response, it is reasonable to believe it can reduce or even eliminate pain associated with fibromyalgia.

Vagus Nerve and Epilepsy

We have been mentioning epilepsy, or seizure disorder, throughout this portion of the book. Namely, because it was the primary disorder that was targeted by vagus nerve stimulation for being able to be cured with the proper techniques. Furthermore, many positive benefits of vagus nerve stimulation were discovered, while researchers were studying the effects of it with epilepsy. Epilepsy is a major central nervous disorder in which brain activity becomes exceedingly abnormal, causing seizures or periods of very unusual behavior. The nerves and neurons are firing uncontrollably, causing erratic and uncontrollable movements. A person who has epilepsy has their whole world turned upside down due to the severity of the condition and the way it takes over their life. A person will often never know when a seizure will hit, which can prevent them from doing many activities like driving. It will also inhibit their ability to go into certain professions. It is a dangerous and stressful disease to have to deal with.

During an epileptic episode, the sympathetic nervous system is incomplete overdrive, causing excessive and erratic movements within the nervous system. When a person is having a full-blown epileptic attack or seizure, we probably won't be able to attempt the many stimulating practices we went over. Much more extreme measures will need to be taken. However, what can be done is the vagal tone can be strengthened to help avoid or reduce epileptic attacks in the future. The stronger the vagal tone, the better adept the parasympathetic response will be, and the better it will become at inhibiting the sympathetic response. We mentioned before how massaging the carotid sinus has been shown to inhibit seizure activity by stimulating the vagus nerve. If this technique can work, then it is a good indication that the other methods will also.

The goal overall is to continuously improve and strengthen the vagus nerve as much as possible. We will not be able to prevent or cure all illnesses. However, as we maintain our own vagal tone, we can help to improve the functionality of the body and at least prevent or reduce many diseases. The point of vagus nerve stimulation is to keep it healthy, active, and strong so that it has the ability to enhance parasympathetic activity as much as possible. When we increase our body's ability to utilize the parasympathetic response, we will be able to reduce seizure activity effectively.

Most of the research behind vagus nerve stimulation has been to help prevent epilepsy. This suggests that it is still considered a strong therapy in inhibiting seizure activity.

Healthy Daily Routines for Vagus Nerve

Regardless of the healthful ampleness of the suppers and tidbits, it is in like manner imperative to counsel with your essential consideration supplier or a Registered Dietitian to assist you with distinguishing nutritional needs altered to you.

Day 1

Breakfast:

1 serving of cereal (½ cup dry oats) arranged with one cup water or skim milk, 1 cut banana, 1 tablespoon of nut spread, and a scramble of cinnamon

Lunch:

1 meal meat move up: Spread mustard on an entire wheat wrap includes four cuts of dish hamburger, four meager cuts of tomatoes, ½ cup of lettuce, and ½ cup of red or green peppers. Firmly fold at that point cut into four equivalent areas.

1 medium banana

Supper:

1 serving of this Greek stuffed peppers formula

1 cup green beans sautéed in a ½ tablespoon of olive oil

Daily Tip:

Make oats medium-term for a speedy, healthy breakfast.

Day 2

Breakfast:

1 veggie omelet, likewise not hesitating to change veggies to preferring

1 cup of blueberries or grapes

Lunch:

1 serving of fish plate of mixed greens: Mix a 5-ounce jar of wild tuna fish with a little avocado, diced carrots and celery, a tablespoon of a lemon squeeze, and salt and pepper to taste. Devour as seems to be, top onto 2 cuts of entire grain bread, or plunge with cut ringer peppers, cucumbers cuts, or carrot sticks

1 medium apple

Supper:

1 side serving of mixed greens with 1 to cups of crude spinach leaves, tomatoes, and cucumber cuts bested with Greek yogurt farm dressing

1 serving eggplant pizza

Daily Tip:

Get the entire family required for a pizza party! Set out irregular fixings and enable them to dress their very own pizza.

Day 3

Breakfast:

1 yogurt-filled melon: Start by on a level plane cut the melon into equal parts. Spoon out the mash and seeds, scoop Greek yogurt into the made "bowl" inside the emptied melon, and sprinkle with ***nuts or seeds for an additional crunch.***

Lunch:

1 turkey sandwich: 2 cuts of entire grain bread, 4 ounces of cut turkey, arranged veggies, as blended greens and cut tomatoes. Smear the bread with 1 tablespoon mustard or olive oil-based mayo.

½ cup curds

½ cup pineapple pieces

Supper:

1 serving mango and avocado plate of mixed greens

2 fish tacos with broccoli slaw

Daily Tip:

Instead of obtaining bundled lunchmeat, get it directly from the butcher in the store to bring down sodium content. Bread is likewise a typical wellspring of sodium, so be watchful for low-sodium brands, or if nothing else providing 140 mg sodium or less per serving.

Day 4

Breakfast:

1 yogurt parfait: 1 cup plain Greek yogurt, 1 cup crisp blueberries, 1 tablespoon cleaved nuts, 1 tablespoon nectar, run of cinnamon

Lunch:

1 serving of cleaved chicken plate of mixed greens: Top three ounces of slashed chicken, two tablespoons of disintegrated low-fat bleu cheddar, ½ cup of hacked cucumbers, 1 tablespoon of hacked walnuts and dried cranberries on 2 cups of a cleaved serving of mixed greens hurled with 2 tablespoons of vinaigrette

1 orange

Supper:

4-ounces simmered turkey bosom

½ cup wild rice and mushroom pilaf

1 cup steamed broccoli

Daily Tip:

After supper, walk the family hound, bicycle around the area, or other physical movement to raise the pulse.

Day 5

Breakfast:

1 serving chocolate banana protein smoothie: Simply consolidate 1 scoop of chocolate protein powder (or enough for 25 to 30 grams of protein), 1 little banana (solidified), ½ cup milk of decision, 1 teaspoon dim chocolate, and ½ cup into a blender and blend until completely joined

Lunch:

1 hot refried dark spicy burro

1 cup cubed watermelon

Supper:

½ cup flame-broiled asparagus

¾ cup flame-broiled potatoes and peppers

1 jalapeno turkey burger

Daily Tip:

Add 1 to 2 tablespoons of chia or flax seeds to the smoothie for included heart-sound fiber and omega-3s.

Day 6

Breakfast:

1 serving high-protein flapjacks, beat with nutty spread, berries, and different top choices

Lunch:

1 serving smooth carrot and sweet potato soup

2 cups blended greens in with 1 cup of favored cleaved veggies (counting broccoli, carrot, and cucumber), 1 tablespoon balsamic vinegar

Supper:

½ cup heated coconut plantains

½ cup dark beans

1 serving pulled pork with salsa verde

Daily Tip:

Appreciate the scraps of the carrot and sweet potato soup by solidifying and warming when prepared to appreciate once more.

Day 7:

Breakfast:

1 avocado egg: Slice avocado into equal parts and take out the enormous pit. Split an egg into the made plunge and heat until the egg whites are cooked and the yolk is at an ideal solidness. Sprinkle on with green onions, diced tomatoes, and a bit of plain Greek yogurt. Shower with hot sauce for a little included zest!

1 navel orange

Lunch:

3-ounces flame-broiled chicken bosom

1 cup of quinoa tabbouleh

Supper:

1 serving Thai salmon bested onto ½ cup dark colored rice

1 cup steamed broccoli

Daily Tip:

Add flavor to the dark-colored rice with minced garlic and other most loved herbs and flavors. Likewise, cook your rice with different veggies for included fiber and micronutrients, alongside making it in enormous clumps for nutritious scraps to begin another week.

Get the nutrients your body needs to function optimally with these recipes that sure to help satiate hunger, keep your gut regular, diminish inflammation, and provide the vitamins and minerals to support a healthy brain, heart, and gut.

Start Your Day: Go Green Smoothie

Begin your day with all the nutrients you need in one quick smoothie!

Serving size: 2 servings

Time: 5 minutes

Ingredients:

- 2 teaspoons lemon juice

- 1 teaspoon peanut butter

- 1 cup unsweetened almond milk

- 2 ounces cucumber

- ½ avocado

- 1 stick celery

- 1 ounce kale leaves

Directions:

1. Toss all ingredients together into a food processor and blitz until smooth and lump-free.

2. Transfer into a glass and enjoy. You can keep the leftovers in a sealed container in the fridge.

3. Tip: Add stevia for sweetness. You can use regular milk in place of the almond milk and any other nut butter in place of peanut butter if you would like.

For the Love of Bread: Keto Bread

Are you trying to stick to a low-carb diet but love bread? Look no further than this light and fluffy keto bread that is delicious served straight from the oven or makes for an excellent slice of toast.

Serving size: 12 slices

Time: 25 minutes

Ingredients:

- 1¼ cups warm water

- Pinch of salt

- 3 teaspoons baking powder

- 1 tablespoon xanthan gum

- 2½ cups almond flour

- 2 cups whey protein

Directions:

1. Mix all your dry ingredients.

2. Gradually add the warm water to this mixture until it is all

evenly combined.

3. Place your mixture into a baking tin that is lined with wax paper.

4. Bake for 20–25 minutes at 375 °F or until you notice the bread has turned a rich golden color.

5. Remove from the oven and let the bread cool down completely before turning it out onto a tray.

6. Enjoy as-is, slice by slice.

Snack Attack: Keto Nut Bar

This is great for a quick breakfast or a snack on the go when feeling hungry.

Serving size: makes about 18 bars

Time: 10 minutes (prep time) and 1 hour (resting time)

Ingredients:

- ¾ cups roasted almonds

- ¾ cups roasted cashew nuts

- 1¼ cups peanuts, salted or unsalted

- Pinch of salt

- 1 teaspoon vanilla extract

- ⅓ cup honey or a substitute

- ½ cup peanut butter

- ¼ cups unsalted butter

Directions:

1. Melt the peanut butter and unsalted butter together in the microwave for one minute.

2. Mix in the honey, salt, and vanilla extract.

3. Add all the nuts into the mixture.

4. Pour this mixture into a wax-paper-lined tray or dish. Evenly spread the mixture.

5. Place the tray or dish into the freezer for one hour or until hard but not frozen solid. You may push down the nuts 30 minutes into the freezing time.

6. Cut into even slices and store them in the fridge.

Breakfast: Berry Boost Keto Pancakes

This recipe is easy to make and delicious!

Serving size: 10

Time: 5 minutes (prep time) and 10 minutes (cook time)

Ingredients:

- A fresh selection of berries, such as raspberries, strawberries, and blueberries

- A handful of chopped pistachios

- A knob of butter to serve and some melted butter for cooking

- ¼ teaspoon baking powder

- 1 teaspoon vanilla essence

- 3 large eggs

- 4.5 ounces cream cheese

- 2.8 ounces (⅔ cup) almond four

Directions:

1. Beat together the cream cheese and flour with a wooden spoon. Slowly beat the eggs into this mixture until smooth and lump-free. Add in the baking powder and vanilla essence.

2. Coat a non-stick pan with melted butter and place this onto a medium heat. Spoon roughly 3¼ cup measures of the batter into the pan and cook until golden brown. Gently turn the pancakes over and cook for a further minute. Move to a plate and continue to cook the rest in this manner.

3. Serve the pancakes with a dash of butter, a handful of pistachios, and a selection of berries.

4. Tip: These are best served warm so that the butter melts right through!

Lunch: Ground-Beef-Filled Cheese Cups

Serve these as an appetizer or a lunchtime meal.

Serving size: 12

Time: 10 minutes (prep time) and 30 minutes (cook time)

Ingredients:

- Extra-virgin olive oil for cooking
- Diced tomatoes
- Chopped cilantro
- 3 minced cloves of garlic
- Chopped avocado
- Dash of sour cream
- Ground black pepper
- *Salt*
- ½ teaspoon paprika
- ½ teaspoon cumin
- 1 teaspoon chili powder
- 1 pound ground beef
- 2 cups grated cheddar cheese
- 1 diced onion

Directions:

1. Heat your oven to 375 °F. Line a large baking tray with a sheet of baking paper. Dish out 2 tablespoons of the cheese onto the tray until the cheese is finished. Be careful to leave

enough space between these mounds so that they do not stick together when melted. Place the tray into the oven and remove once the cheese has melted and turned a golden-brown color around the edges. This will take roughly 6 minutes or so. Leave to cool for 1 minute.

2. Grease the bottom of a muffin tray with cooking spray. Gently place the cheese spheres over the bottom of the muffin tray. Place another muffin tray over the bottom of the first muffin tin, thus shaping the cheese into "cup" shapes. Let cool for 10 minutes. If you do not own a second muffin tray, you can easily use your hands to mold the cheese into "cup" shapes.

3. Over medium heat, add olive oil and fry the diced onion until soft and translucent. Next, add the ground beef and garlic. Mix it up with a wooden spoon until cooked through and the meat is evenly browned. Drain off any unwanted fat.

4. Add the salt, pepper, chili powder, cumin, and paprika. Give the mixture a good final stir and set it aside.

5. By now, you will have perfectly molded cheese cups. Place the cups on a serving tray. Fill them with the beef mixture.

6. Top the cups with a dash of sour cream, chopped avo, and tomato. Finish off with a pinch of cilantro.

Dinner: Coconut Chicken Curry

In under an hour, you can serve up a super supper for the whole family. This recipe is both gluten-free and keto-friendly.

Serving size: 4 servings

Time: 20 minutes (prep time) and 25 minutes (cook time)

Ingredients:

- Olive oil

- Fish sauce

- Fresh lime juice

- 1 teaspoon ground coriander

- 2 teaspoons ground cumin

- ½ teaspoon turmeric

- 2 teaspoons mustard seeds

- 2 chopped red chilies

- 2 teaspoons fresh ginger

- 2 crushed cloves of garlic

- Olive oil

- 1.3 pounds chicken thigh fillets, chopped into pieces of 1–1.5 inches

- 1 onion

- 400 milliliters coconut cream

- 3.5 ounces baby spinach leaves

- 18 ounces chopped broccoli

Directions:

1. Over high heat, add oil to a large saucepan. Add half the chicken pieces until evenly browned. Remove from heat and do the same with the remainder of the chicken. Set all the chicken aside.

2. Add a dash of oil to the saucepan. Add the onion until softened. Add your spices, coriander, cumin, chili, garlic, ginger, mustard seeds, and turmeric. Cook through for 2 minutes, stirring occasionally.

3. Add the coconut cream and chicken to the onion and spice mixture. Bring to a boil. Slowly reduce the heat to a simmer. Partially cover the saucepan with a lid. Let the mixture simmer for a further 20 minutes or until the chicken is tender and cooked through.

4. Process the broccoli in a food processor until it looks like rice. Add this to a microwave-safe dish and cover. For 2–3 minutes, microwave on high.

5. Remove the coconut chicken curry and serve over the broccoli rice. Add a dash of freshly squeezed lime juice and fish sauce to taste. Top with spinach and extra chili for added zing!

Dessert: Ice Cream

What would a meal be without dessert?

Serving size: 8 servings

Time: Approximately 8 hours

Ingredients:

- Fresh berries

- Cocoa powder

- Pinch of salt

- 1 teaspoon vanilla essence

- ¼ cup swerve confectioners sweetener

- 2 cups heavy cream

- 15 ounces (2 cans) coconut cream

Directions:

1. Chill coconut cream overnight.

2. Dish out the coconut cream, leaving the liquid behind. Using a hand mixer, beat the coconut cream until thick and creamy. Set this aside.

3. In a separate bowl, beat the heavy cream into soft peaks. Add

the salt, vanilla essence, and sweetener.

4. Fold in the heavy cream and coconut cream.

5. Transfer the cream mixture into a bread tin.

6. Place in the freezer for 5 hours or until firm.

7. Serve with a dash of berries and a dusting of cocoa powder.

8. Tip: The ice cream can prove a bit tough to dish up. It is suggested that you let it thaw for a few minutes. You can keep the leftover coconut water from the tin and use it in a smoothie as an alternative to throwing it away.

CHAPTER 7

Vagus Nerve and Social Engangement Learning

Our Autonomic Nervous System (ANS), is the director of the internal symphony in our body. It is liable for the control of our real capacities not intentionally coordinated, for example, breathing, the heartbeat, pulse, sweating, and related stomach procedures. The ANS is continually murmuring at a specific beat, and how well it works determines our physical, mental, and enthusiastic well-being.

The Social Engagement System

The Vagus Nerve is related to increments in wellbeing and passionate prosperity as it produces favorable conditions of unwinding and social commitment. Our Social Engagement framework is working ideally when we have a sense of security and associate with the world and others. For the day, we always get signs and triggers through our faculties and sash, which acts as a second sensory system.

We have an extreme situation, which is the outside world. Yet, we additionally have an inward domain, which is the physiology of our body, such as jumping into a remote ocean, so much is occurring underneath the surface, and wave after wave.

Our intuitive inside sifting framework will promptly assess whether we are sheltered or need to make a move. This occurs without us in any event, monitoring it, or contemplating it. When we have a sense of security, we can unwind, grow, go ahead, and step into the world. When there is pressure or apparent risk in our psyches, we depend on our social commitment framework to set up a feeling of wellbeing and association. This can be accomplished through a discussion, a call for help, looking, or hearing a quieting voice. This will send flags down to our hearts and lungs, hindering our pulse and extending our relaxing. It mostly works as a foot brake - a Vagal Brake - and has a quieting and alleviating impact on our sensory system.

Picture the inverse: For instance, an individual says something to you that makes you feel upset. What occurs? We will generally change our outward appearance flagging our agitated, the tone of our voice changes frequently to an angrier, more robust, or higher pitch. We look for approval, and we get the telephone and converse with somebody. On the off chance that the social commitment framework neglects to determine the pressure and it stays dynamic in our body, at that point we will naturally turn to the more established organic reaction, one stage down the stepping stool into battle/flight, with the Sympathetic Nervous framework kicking in.

Diseases Associated with Vagus Nerve

What's Anxiety?

Anxiety is your body's response to harmful situations - whether perceived or real. When you feel endangered, a chemical reaction happens in the human body, which lets you behave in a way that reduces harm. This response is called "fight-or-flight," and also even the stress reaction. During a stress reaction, your heart rate increases, breathing accelerates, muscles tighten, and blood pressure increases. You have gotten prepared to behave. It is the way you protect yourself.

Anxiety affects all of us. You will detect anxiety symptoms if you are disciplining your children through busy days at work, handling your finances, or dealing with a problematic relationship. Anxiety is everywhere. And if a tiny strain is OK - a little stress is really beneficial - a lot of anxiety can put you back down and make you ill, both emotionally and physically.

The very first step to controlling anxiety is to be aware of the signs of anxiety. But recognizing anxiety symptoms could be more complicated than you might imagine. The majority of us are used to being worried, and we frequently don't understand we're worried until we're at the breaking point.

Stress means different things to various men and women. What causes anxiety in one person could be of no concern to the next. Some folks are much better able to manage stress than many others. And, not all stress is bad. In tiny doses, anxiety can help you achieve activities and keep you from getting hurt. For instance, anxiety is what makes you hit the brakes to avoid hitting the vehicle in front of you. That is a fantastic thing.

Our bodies were created to manage small doses of anxiety. However, we're not equipped to take care of long-term, chronic pressure without ill effects.

The Effects of Chronic Anxiety

Your nervous system is not very good at differentiating between psychological and physical dangers. If you are super stressed within a debate with a buddy, a job deadline, or even a mountain of invoices, your body is able to respond as strongly as though you're confronting an authentic life-or-death circumstance. The longer your emergency pressure process is triggered, the easier it becomes a trigger, which makes it more challenging.

If you tend to get stressed out often, like most people in the demanding world, the human body can exist at a heightened state of anxiety the majority of the time. And that may result in serious health issues. Chronic stress disrupts just about any system in human life. It may suppress your immune system, upsets your digestive and reproductive processes, raises the probability of heart attack and stroke, obesity, and accelerates the aging procedure. It may even rewire the mind, which makes you vulnerable to stress, depression, and other mental health issues.

Health issues caused or Exacerbated by anxiety include:

- Anxiety and stress

- Anxiety of some sort

- Sleep issues

- Autoimmune diseases

- Esophageal issues

- Skin problems, including psoriasis

- Heart disorder

- Weight issues

- Reproductive problems

- Memory and immune issues

Signs and Symptoms of Anxiety Overload

The most damaging thing about worry is how easily it can creep up on you. You become accustomed to it. It begins to feel comfortable, even ordinary. You do not notice just how much it is bothering you personally, even as it requires a hefty toll. That is why it's essential to know about the frequent warning signs and symptoms of pressure overload.

Emotional symptoms:

- Memory issues

- Inability to focus

- Poor conclusion

- Seeing just the unwanted

- Anxious or rushing ideas

- Continuous stressing

Psychological symptoms:

- Anxiety or overall unhappiness

- Stress and burnout

- Moodiness, irritability, or anger

- Feeling overwhelmed

- Loneliness and isolation

- Other psychological or psychological health issues

Physical signs:

- Aches and pains

- Diarrhea or constipation

- Nausea, nausea

- Abdominal pain, fast heartbeat

- reduction of sexual drive

- Frequent colds or influenza

Possible symptoms:

- Eating less or more

- Sleeping too much or too small

- Withdrawing from the others

- Procrastinating or failing responsibilities

- Utilizing alcohol, smoking cigarettes, or medications to

unwind

- Nervous habits (e.g. nail biting)

Reasons Of Anxiety

The scenarios and anxieties that cause anxiety are called stressors. We usually consider stressors as being unwanted, including an exhausting job program or even a rocky relationship. But whatever sets high requirements on you can cause you to be more stressed. Including festive events like getting married, purchasing a home, moving to school, or getting a promotion.

Not all stress is due to outside elements. Anxiety may also be inner or self-generated, i.e., if you worry too about something which might or might not occur, or possess absurd, pessimistic notions about life.

Where one individual thrives under pressure and also plays well on the surface of a tight deadline, then another will close down if work needs escalate. And as you will delight in helping to look after your older parents, your sisters might find the requirements of caretaking overpowering and overwhelming.

Frequent Outside Triggers of Anxiety Include:

- Significant life changes

- Function or college

- Relationship problems

- Fiscal problems

- Being overly active

- Kids and household

Frequent Inner Triggers of Anxiety Include:

- Pessimism
- Inability to take doubt
- Rigid thinking, insufficient versatility
- Negative Allergic
- Unrealistic expectations / perfectionism
- All-or-nothing mindset

How Much Pressure Is too much?

Due to the widespread harm stress can trigger, it is crucial that you learn your limitation. But exactly how much pressure is "a lot" differs from person to person. Many people today appear to have the ability to roll with life's thoughts, but some have a tendency to crumble in the face of minor hurdles or frustrations. Some individuals thrive on the enthusiasm of a high-stress way of life.

Factors which Affect your Anxiety Tolerance Level Comprise:

- Your service community. A powerful network of supportive family and friends members is a tremendous barrier against stress. Whenever you have people you can depend on, life stresses do not appear too overwhelming. On the reverse side, the lonelier and more isolated you are, the higher your chance of succumbing to pressure.

- Your awareness of management. If you have confidence in your ability to affect events and innovate through challenges, it is simpler to keep anxiety in stride. On the other hand, if you think you have very little control over your lifetime and are at the mercy of the surroundings and conditions, anxiety is much more likely to knock you off track.

- Your mindset and outlook. How you see life and its inescapable struggles makes a massive difference in your ability to deal with stress. If you are normally hopeful and optimistic, you will be somewhat vulnerable. Stress-hardy men and women have a tendency to embrace struggles, have a more powerful sense of comedy, believe in a greater goal, and take change as an unavoidable part of existence.

- Your capacity to take care of your feelings. If you do not find out how to unwind and soothe yourself if you are feeling depressed, upset, or upset, you are more likely to worry and be stressed even over the smallest bad things that occur in life. Possessing the capacity to recognize and deal appropriately with your feelings will boost your tolerance to stress and also allow you to bounce back from hardship.

- Your wisdom and prep. The more you understand about a stressful position, for example, how much time it will last and what to anticipate, the simpler it is to deal with it. By way of instance, if you go into an operation with a realistic image of what to expect post-op, a debilitating recovery will be less stressful than if you're hoping to bounce back fast.

Improving your Capacity to Manage Anxiety

- Get going. Upping your activity level is one strategy you'll be able to use immediately to help alleviate strain and begin to feel much better. Routine exercise can raise your mood and also function as a diversion from stresses, letting you break from this cycle of unwanted thoughts that nourish anxiety. Rhythmic exercises like walking, jogging, swimming, and dance are incredibly successful, particularly in the event you exercise mindfully (focusing your attention on the physical sensations you encounter as you proceed)

- Thus, spend some time with individuals who enhance your disposition and do not allow your duties to keep you from having a social life. If you do not have any intimate relationships or your relationships are the source of the anxiety, make it a priority to construct more effective and more fulfilling relationships.

- Engage your perceptions. Another quick method to alleviate anxiety is by engaging at least one of your perceptions --sight, sound, taste, odor, touch, or motion. The crucial thing is to obtain the sensory input that is effective for you. Does listening to an uplifting tune cause you to feel calm? Or smelling black coffee? Or perhaps petting animal functions fast to cause you to feel focused? Everyone reacts to sensory input differently, and you should experiment to discover what works better for you.

- Learn how to unwind. You cannot altogether remove stress from your daily life, but you can control just how much it impacts you. Comfort techniques like meditation, yoga, and deep breathing trigger your body's relaxation response, a state of restfulness that's the polar opposite of this stress reaction. When practiced often, these actions can lessen your daily stress levels and enhance feelings of pleasure and calmness. They also raise your ability to remain calm under pressure.

- Eat a nutritious diet. The foods you consume can worsen or improve your mood and influence your ability to deal with life's frustrations. Eating a diet filled with processed and convenience foods, processed carbohydrates, and sugary snacks may aggravate anxiety symptoms, even though a diet full of fresh vegetables and fruit, high-quality protein, and omega-3 fatty acids, can help you cope with life's ups and downs.

- Get your rest. Feeling drained can boost stress by inducing one to think irrationally. At precisely the same time, chronic anxiety can interrupt your sleep. Whether you are having difficulty falling asleep or remaining asleep through the nighttime, there are tons of approaches to enhance your sleeping so that you feel less anxious, more effective and mentally balanced.

Autonomic Dysfunction

The (ANS) controls several primary functions, such as:

- Heart Speed

- Body Temperature

- Breathing Speed

- Digestion

- Sense

You do not need to think consciously about those systems to allow them to get the job done. The ANS provides the link between your brain and particular body components, such as internal organs.

The primary responsibility of the SANS is to activate emergency responses if required. All these fight-or-flight responses make you prepared to react to stressful scenarios. The PANS boost your energy and also calms cells for everyday functions.

Autonomic Dysfunction

Autonomic dysfunction can vary in symptoms and seriousness, and they frequently stem from various underlying causes. Some kinds of adrenal dysfunction can be quite abrupt and intense but are additionally reversible.

Autonomic dysfunction develops when the nerves of the ANS are damaged. This problem is known as adrenal disorder or dysautonomia.

Autonomic dysfunction may vary from moderate to life-threatening. It may impact a portion of the ANS or even the whole ANS. On occasion, the ailments that cause difficulties are temporary and reversible. Others have been chronic, or of long duration, and might continue to worsen as time passes.

Diabetes, along with Parkinson's disorder, have been two cases of chronic illnesses that may result in autonomic dysfunction.

Symptoms of Adrenal Dysfunction

Some signs that may signal the existence of an adrenal nerve disease include:

- Nausea and fainting upon standing up, or orthostatic hypotension

- A inability to change heartbeat with exercise, or exercise deprivation

- Sweat abnormalities, that may switch between sweating too much rather than sweating sufficiently

- Gastrointestinal troubles, like a reduction of desire, bloating, nausea, constipation, or even trouble swallowing

Various Kinds of Autonomic Dysfunction:

Postural orthostatic tachycardia Infection (POTS)

POTS affects a large amount of the overall population, from 1 to 3 million individuals in the USA only. Almost five times more women have this illness in contrast to guys. It may affect children, teens, and adults.

POTS symptoms may vary from moderate to severe. As much as one in four individuals with POTS have considerable limitations in action and cannot work because of their affliction.

Neurocardiogenic syncope (NCS)

NCS can also be called vasovagal syncope. It is a typical source of syncope or fainting. The fainting is due to a sudden slowing of blood circulation into the brain. It may be actuated with dehydration, standing, or sitting for quite a very long time, a warm environment and stressful feelings. People frequently have nausea, sweat, excessive fatigue, and sick feelings before and following an episode.

Multiple system atrophy (MSA)

MSA is a deadly kind of adrenal dysfunction. Early on, its symptoms are very similar to Parkinson's disease. But individuals with this condition usually have a life expectancy of just about 5 to ten years after diagnosis. It is a rare illness that typically occurs in adults over age 40. The reason behind MSA is unknown and without a treatment or cure for the illness.

Hereditary sensory and sensory neuropathies (HSAN)

HSAN is a set of associated genetic disorders which lead to widespread nerve disorder in children and adults. The status may result in an inability to sense pain, temperature fluctuations, as well as touch. Additionally, it may impact a vast array of body functions. The disease is categorized into four distinct groups based on age, inherited routines, and even symptoms.

Holmes-Adie syndrome (HAS)

HAS mostly affects the nerves controlling the muscles of the eye, resulting in vision issues. One pupil will probably be more prominent than another, and it'll constrict gradually in a glowing light. Frequently it includes both eyes. Deep tendon reflexes, such as those from the Achilles tendon, might likewise be absent.

HAS may happen because of a viral infection, which leads to swelling and swelling neurons. The loss of deep tendon reflexes is irreversible, but HAN is not considered life-threatening. Eyeglasses and drops can help fix vision problems.

Other kinds of adrenal dysfunction can lead to illness or harm to your physique. Autonomic neuropathy describes damage to nerves in specific medicines, trauma, or illness. Some ailments causing this disease include:

- Uncontrolled elevated blood pressure

- Long-term heavy drinking

- Diabetes

- Autoimmune ailments

Your physician will treat autonomic malfunction by fixing the indicators. When an underlying illness is causing the issue, it is important to get it under control whenever possible.

Orthostatic Intolerance

Orthostatic intolerance is a condition wherever your system is influenced by changes in place. A vertical position causes symptoms of nausea, lightheadedness, nausea, perspiration, and tingling. Slimming down enhances the indicators. Frequently this is related to an improper regulation of the ANS.

Other kinds of orthostatic Intolerance include:

- Postural orthostatic tachycardia syndrome

- Neurocardiogenic syncope or vasovagal syncope

How is Adrenal Dysfunction Handled?

Your Physician will treat autonomic Malfunction by fixing the indicators. When an underlying illness is causing the issue, it is important to get it under control whenever possible.

Frequently, it may be aided by lifestyle modifications and prescription drugs. The outward symptoms can react to:

- Enhancing the head of your mattress

- Drinking sufficient fluids

- Adding salt to a daily diet

- Sporting compression sleeves to avoid blood pooling in your legs

- Altering positions gradually

- Taking drugs ,including midodrine

- Nerve damage is tough to heal. Physical treatment, walking aids, feeding tubes, and other techniques could be essential to assist in treating more acute nerve involvement.

Depression and Nervousness

Anxiety and depression are distinct circumstances, but they generally occur together. Besides, they have comparable therapies.

Feeling down or feeling the blues today is normal. And everybody feels anxious from time to time. It's a normal reaction to stressful circumstances. But acute or continuing feelings of depression and stress may indicate an underlying mental health condition.

Stress can occur as a symptom of clinical (major) depression) Additionally, it is normal to have depression that is triggered by means of an anxiety disorder, like generalized anxiety disorder, anxiety disorder or separation anxiety disorder. A lot of individuals have an identification of an anxiety disorder and clinical depression.

Indicators of both ailments usually are helped with emotional counseling (psychotherapy), drugs, like antidepressants, or even both. Lifestyle modifications, like improving sleep habits, increasing social assistance, utilizing stress-reduction tactics, or getting regular exercise, can also help. In case you have either illness, avoid smoking, smoking, and psychiatric medication. They could make both circumstances worse and interfere with therapy.

Depression and Stress: How to Recognize and Treat Coexisting Infection

Anxiety and depression can happen at the exact identical moment. In reality, it's been projected that 45 percentage of individuals with one psychological health state meet the standards for a couple of disorders.

Though each state has its very own triggers, they can share similar symptoms and remedies. Keep reading to find out, including getting strategies for direction and what to anticipate from a medical investigation.

What Are the Signs of each Illness?

Some signs of depression and anxiety overlap, like difficulties with sleep, irritability, depression, and trouble concentrating. However there are many important differences which help differentiate between both.

Depression

Feeling down, sad, or angry is normal. It may be about feeling that way for many days or months on end.

Physical signs and behavioral changes brought on by depression comprise:

- Diminished energy, chronic fatigue, or feeling lethargic frequently

- Trouble concentrating, making decisions, or remembering

- Pain, aches, aches, or gastrointestinal troubles with no obvious cause

- Fluctuations in appetite or weight

- Trouble sleeping, waking early, or oversleeping

Emotional Signs of Depression Comprise:

- Reduction of interest or some more finding enjoyment in hobbies or activities

- Persistent feelings of sadness, anxiety, or bitterness

- Feeling hopeless or pessimistic

- Anger, irritability, or restlessness

- Feeling guilty or undergoing feelings of worthlessness or feedback

- Ideas of suicide or death

- Suicide efforts

- Stress

Stress, or anxiety and nervousness, can happen to anybody from time to time. It is not uncommon to experience stress prior to a huge event or a significant choice.

However, chronic stress could be painful and lead to irrational ideas and fears that interfere with your everyday life.

Physical signs and behavioral changes brought on by generalized anxiety disorder comprise:

- Feeling exhausted easily

- Trouble concentrating or remembering

- Muscle strain

- Fast heartrate

- Jagged teeth

- Sleep problems, such as difficulties falling asleep and restless, unsatisfying sleep

Psychological symptoms of stress comprise:

- Restlessness, irritability, or feeling on edge

- Trouble commanding fear or anxiety

- Fear

A Self-Help Test Might Help you Determine the Indications

You know what is normal for you. If you end up experiencing feelings or behaviours that are not typical or when something sounds off, this may be an indication you will want to seek out assistance from a health care provider. It is always preferable to chat about what you are experiencing and feeling in order that treatment can start early if it's needed.

With that said, some online self-diagnosis evaluations are readily available to assist you understand what could be occurring. These evaluations, while useful, are not a replacement for an expert diagnosis from your physician. They cannot take different ailments which could be impacting your wellbeing into consideration, either.

Popular self-help evaluations for stress and depression comprise:

- Depression test and stress evaluation

- Depression evaluation

- Stress evaluation

The Way To Handle your Symptoms

Besides a proper therapy strategy from your physician, these plans might help you find relief from your symptoms. It is essential to understand. However, these hints might not work for everybody, and they might not work every time.

The objective of treating depression and stress is to produce several treatment choices which may all work together to aid, to an extent, whenever you want to use them.

Allow yourself to feel that which you are feeling -- and also understand that it is not your fault.

Anxiety and anxiety disorders are all medical ailments. They are not a consequence of weakness or failure. What you believe is the result of inherent causes and causes; it isn't the consequence of something that you did or did not do.

Do something that you have control over, such as making your bed or carrying out the garbage. At the moment, regaining a little power or management can help you deal with overwhelming symptoms. Accomplish a job you're able to handle, like neatly restacking publications or sorting out your recycling.

Do something to give yourself a feeling of achievement and energy.

You May also create a morning, day, or regular daily activity. Regular activity is occasionally useful for individuals with depression and anxiety. This gives structure and a feeling of control. Additionally, it lets you make space in your daily life for self-care techniques, enabling you to control the symptoms.

Do your best to adhere to some sleep program. Aim to get seven to eight hours per night. Less or more than this will complicate symptoms of conditions. Insufficient or inadequate sleep may cause issues with your own cardiovascular, endocrine, immune, and nervous disorders.

Attempt to eat something healthy, like an apple or some nuts, at least once each day. If you are feeling miserable or stressed, you might reach for soothing foods such as sweets and pasta to relieve some of the strain. Nonetheless, these foods offer little nutrition. Try to help nourish your using vegetables, fruits, lean meats, and whole grains.

If you are up for it, then go for a walk around the block. Exercise may be an effective remedy for depression since it is a natural mood booster that releases feel-good hormones. But for many individuals, a gym may cause anxiety and anxiety. If that is true for you, start looking for more natural approaches to use, like walking around your area or searching for an Internet exercise movie you can perform in the home.

Do something which you know brings you relaxation, like seeing a favorite film or writing in a journal.

Give yourself time to focus on you, along with the things you prefer. Downtime is an excellent way to allow your body to rest, and it may distract your brain with things that bring you an increase in energy.

In case you haven't left home in some time, look at doing whatever you find calming, such as getting your nails done or obtaining a massage.

Relaxation techniques may enhance your wellbeing and might lessen symptoms of depression and nervousness.

Find an action that feels appropriate for you, and you can frequently exercise, for example:

- Yoga

- Meditation

- Breathing exercises

- Massage

Reach out to someone you are comfortable speaking to and speak about anything you want, like how you are feeling or talk about anything you watched on Twitter.

Healthy relationships are just one of the best approaches that will assist you in feeling much better. Connecting using a buddy or relative could offer a natural boost and permit you to locate a trusted supply of encouragement and support.

What are the Zones Innervated by the Ventral Vagus Nerve?

The Ventral Vagus Nerve innervates the territories over the stomach: face, throat, voice box, larynx, center ear, heart, lungs, and serves the social commitment framework. Five cranial nerves manage this framework, and when these nerves work well, we can appreciate ideal physical and enthusiastic wellbeing, including extraordinary companionship, backing, holding, and adoring connections. At the point when we are socially drawn in, we can be inventive, joyful, gainful, and upbeat.

Socially connected implies we are free from dangers, peril, superfluous stresses, and now in extraordinary physical wellbeing. The Social Engagement System guides us in direction, correspondence, and outward appearance and involves the accompanying cranial nerves, which all begin in the brainstem.

5th Cranial Nerve: this is the Trigeminal Nerve: it is the face and jaw biting muscles.

7th Cranial Nerve: this is the Facial Nerve: it controls hearing, center ear, and every facial muscle for informative outward appearances and copy. Neural guideline for the center ear muscles

9th Cranial Nerve: this is Glossopharyngeal Nerve: it controls the Tongue, Throat, and Swallowing. It is answerable for sounds delivered by the Voicebox, vocal tone, and making sounds.

10th Cranial Nerve: this is the Ventral Vagus Nerve branch. It innervates little muscles in the throat and salivation.

11th Cranial Nerve: it innervates the Trapezius and Sternocleidomastoid (SCM) muscles in the neck for head and neck development, direction, and having the option to turn your head.

<u>Practices we Show when Socially Engaged:</u>

- We have a sense of security

- We are associated with ourselves and to other people,

- We can be close

- We contact an associate with others, we can bond

- We are quiet, inhale effectively, and we can think unmistakably

- Muscles are loose

- We feel fun-loving, we move, sing and tummy chuckle

- We feel love and can really cherish

- We can really unwind and unwind into association with others

- Feel the world: it is wide, and we are one with the surroundings

Side Effects We Can Have when not Socially Locked in:

- We feel on edge or are not ready to unwind around ourselves as well as other people

- We feel shut down or discouraged

- We are overpowered

- We feel outraged, nauseate, disgrace

- We habitually need to do things

- We are wired

- We are antisocial people - don't generally draw in and escape the world

Craniosacral Therapy

The craniosacral system comprises of the film encompassing the spinal string, spinal liquid, the spinal string sac, and the mind. Alongside the focal sensory system, this framework is the most powerful framework contained inside the human body.

The spinal rope and the cerebrum contained inside this framework, impact, and help control the focal sensory system. The two frameworks together control body development, perception, thinking, feelings, and wellbeing. When there is a glitch in this framework, the wellbeing of the whole body is in peril.

The spinal liquid that is contained inside the film, known as the meninges, beats at a particular cadence for every individual. As a rule, this spinal liquid heartbeat rate is around ten heartbeats for each moment. This craniosacral beat is like circulatory strain, in that it beats as it moves, both all through the spinal string. Any damage can make the pressure be put on the liquid and can interfere with the equalization of the spinal liquid stream.

Whenever the liquid is blocked or can't beat accurately, medical issues are framed. Weight put on the spinal fluid can influence the whole body and cause hurts, torments, problems concentrating, limited development, and different issues, for example, migraines, ceaseless exhaustion disorder, fibromyalgia, scoliosis, and other connective tissue and joint sicknesses.

What is Craniosacral Therapy?

Most researchers structured craniosacral treatment during the 1970s. He put together his way to deal with recuperation, with respect to standards and hypotheses made by some researchers, who was a rehearsing osteopath during the 1900s. Dr. Upledger went through years rehearsing and consummating his system. Upledger, a biomechanics teacher at Michigan State University, held great and several clinical preliminaries as he dealt with this new method for recuperating.

The rule behind CST is the information on how the spinal

framework functions and how the power behind the recuperating parts likewise. Regular stressors can affect the weight of the spinal liquid, just as mishaps and damage. By utilizing a light touch, experts of CST can frequently get the liquids streaming and beating in an ordinary way, thus facilitating the torments that a blocked stream can cause.

Likewise, CST can discharge pressures and stressors that are contained in the tissues encompassing the framework. This way helps keep up with the spinal and cerebrum framework; however, it can likewise work to fix the focal sensory system. By normalizing the beats and the rhythms of the cerebrospinal liquid around the spine and the cerebrum, dysfunctions of the body, for example, continuous agony, strokes, neurological hindrances, and sports wounds can be both reduced and restored.

What are Craniosacral Therapy Benefits?

- Headaches and Chronic headaches

- Chronic neck torment

- Upper and lower-back agony

- Stress and pressure

- Chronic weariness disorder

- Fibromyalgia

- Post-horrendous pressure disorder

- Orthopedic issues

- Arthritis

Moreover, great people discover that the treatment is incredibly unwinding. Numerous individuals will, in general float off to rest during their treatment. This is, in reality, exceptionally helpful because a casual body reacts better to remedial recuperating.

Different advantages incorporate the impact it has on the connective tissues of the body. These connective tissues cannot just apply excessive weight on the muscles, but they likewise can restrain movement. Since they are not ready to be seen on most analytic pictures, the manifestations an individual display can frequently appear to be strange and are regularly rejected by conventional therapeutic professionals.

Another part of CST is Somato-Emotional Release, which holds that feelings are additionally part of a bodily injury and that by discharging the horrible feelings, mending is quicker and progressively successful. Regularly, the back-rub systems utilized in the CST discharges these feelings. Other treatment benefits incorporate mindfulness of the body and the arrival of the body's oblivious recuperating capacities.

Typically, the customer or patient rests completely dressed on an agreeable couch or unique remedial table. The Craniosacral Therapist, at that point, tenderly lays their hands on the patient. Most of the craniosacral advisors are osteopaths, chiropractors, rub specialists, or physical advisors.

Subsequent to getting a full restorative history from the customer, the advisor at that point starts with the feet. Utilizing a lightweight, close to the weight applied by a coin being set on the skin, the specialist begins to stir their way up the body of the patient. For the most part, the advisor begins with the feet and works upwards. Notwithstanding, utilizing CST, applied kinesiology, is likewise used to help with the reflexive methodology.

CST is a comprehensive treatment since it attempts to avoid and fix ailment and malady by utilizing the body in general. Specialists who practice CST are commonly delicate professionals who tune in to their patients.

CHAPTER 8

Chronic inflammation

When the vagus nerve is not functioning correctly, one of the first hints is the inability of the body to manage inflammation properly. It means the vagus nerve is not effectively doing its job, which is to act as a message network between the immune system and the brain. Many factors can cause inflammation. That is why experts rarely look at the vagus nerve. Inflammation can be corrected only when we find out what was responsible for it.

Inflammation may be mild, and we know that inflammation is the body's way of defending itself. Inflammation becomes a health problem when it becomes chronic.

Chronic inflammation can manifest itself physically in many ways, from cancer to autoimmune diseases, growth of a tumor, and arthritis.

Inflammation becomes chronic due to the inability of the vagus nerve to transmit the signals required to stop inflammation. You can try to stimulate the vagus nerve and improve the vagal tone. This enhances the vagus nerve's ability to transmit signals between the white blood cells and the brain. Effective signaling from the vagus nerve will reverse inflammation without the need for any medication. Then the body can try to repair the damaged cells.

Some of the most common inflammation is caused by physical and emotional trauma.

These are chronic inflammation of the gut and autoimmune conditions.

Inflammation Caused by Physical and Emotional Trauma

Physical traumas cause the most apparent types of inflammation. When you sprain an ankle or bump a body part, it soon becomes red, swollen, and sore. This is due to the actions of the white blood cells. The cells increase blood flow and secretion to chemicals to the spot to repair the damage and fight any invading pathogen. These symptoms are only supposed to exist for a short period of time, pending the time that the body heals itself. When they remain, it starts to harm the body. It means the cholinergic anti-inflammatory pathway (which acts as a signal network between the antibodies) and the vagus nerve has failed in their task of transmitting the information.

There are various reasons for inflammation to remain over a longer than normal period of time. All these reasons prevent the body from healing correctly.

One curveball responsible for inflammation is emotional trauma. This stress applied to the mind can create a negative attitude that affects one's perception of the environment and other people. Emotional trauma may vary in severity and the impact on the individual. The effect of emotional trauma can also be affected by the number of emotionally traumatic events and how closely together they happen.

It is easier for us to recover from things that happened a few years apart than for something that happened a few days apart.

Emotionally traumatic events trigger the sympathetic forces that put us in fight or flight mode. This increases the likeliness of inflammation and reduces the ability of the vagus nerve to stop inflammation.

Emotional trauma rarely acts alone. It combines with physical trauma (the quick and ready cause of inflammation) to form a deadly combination. The actions of the emotional trauma expand any inflammation from physical trauma.

In the end, inflammation becomes chronic, and more complicated health problems start to rear their heads. Much like the way chronic stress works, small physical trauma can lead to more complicated health problems, because numerous other emotional and physical trauma have complicated the parasympathetic nerves of the vagus nerve.

Chronic Inflammation of the Gut

The white blood cells can become desensitized to inflammation if inflammation repeatedly occurs over a long period of time. The white blood cells are the little soldiers of the body. They protect it. Constant inflammation will impact them negatively.

Inflammation in the gut is a tricky situation because we can't quickly identify the symptoms. It doesn't manifest externally until the problem becomes really severe. You can find a test online or visit your health provider.

An imbalance in the digestive tract's microbiome population is the most common factor responsible for inflammation in the gut. There are other causes, such as the consumption of inflammatory food items, but the one mentioned above is the most rampant.

It is not just the white blood cells and antibodies that can get desensitized to inflammation. Constant inflammation can also wear out the vagus nerve. It begins to learn to ignore inflammatory signals, which results in a disastrous situation because it misses its job, which is to send alerts to the antibodies to stop inflammation. When it doesn't do its job, the inflammation won't stop, and the antibodies will start to attack healthy cells of the body.

Young people are relatively safe, but inflammation begins to get worse after you reach 30 years of age. The functionality of the vagus nerve and vagal tone has reduced significantly. It has learned over the years to ignore inflammatory symptoms and signals. It not just age that minimizes the influence of the vagus nerve and vagal tone on inflammation, other situations that put people in delicate health conditions can also cause it. Examples include pregnancy and childbirth, sickness and emotional trauma.

Autoimmune Conditions

Chronic stress, our lifestyle and poor dietary choices contribute to autoimmune conditions. It is one of the most rapidly growing health conditions in the United States. Examples of autoimmune health conditions include rheumatoid arthritis, alopecia areata, Graves' disease, Hashimoto's thyroiditis, psoriasis, multiple sclerosis, Crohn's disease, systemic lupus erythematosus, type 1 diabetes and celiac disease, and many others. There is much more where that comes from.

Most of these health conditions start in the digestive tract, which is fitting because it contains the largest population of immune cells. These cells are located here in large quantities because it is also the point of access into the body for many toxins, pathogens, and chemicals. The other end of access is broken skin, but it is not nearly as porous as the mouth and digestive tract.

The immune cells are lined along the walls of the digestive tract. They are held in lymphatic tissues built like pocket spaces called GALT.

The immune cells of the digestive tract encounter numerous invaders which they are there to fight against. The persistent entrance of these invading toxins and pathogens can desensitize the immune cells to them. Over a long period of time, they begin to stop reacting to and fighting the invaders. They have worked so hard that they have become third. This is how autoimmune problems start.

Some autoimmune diseases are hereditary, but it still requires to be triggered.

The Factors that Contribute to the Risk of Developing an Autoimmune Disease:

-   An amount of autoimmune, autoreactive T cells in the GALT

-   An imbalance in the gut microbiome that is pro-inflammation

-   Hereditary genes that are susceptible to autoimmune conditions

There isn't much we can do about the first and last factors. We don't know the amount of autoimmune cells in the GALT, we also can't change our genes. What we can do is to influence the second factor, the balance of microbiome in the gut. We can do this by feeding the microbiome with the right food items.

Post-Traumatic Stress Disorder (PTSD)

Post-traumatic stress disorder (PTSD) first came to public attention after World War 1, then it was called shell shock, and the public was divided over it. There is barely any division on PTSD's legality as a medical condition today, which is a good thing. The bad part is that PTSD has become more common in our society. Many people today are suffering from PTSD, far more than you would think because most people expect only soldiers and armed combatants to be who have PTSD, but anyone who has been subjected to a traumatic event can suffer from PTSD.

The Autonomic Nervous System and Trauma

The autonomic nervous system is very resilient and can quickly recover from many events. Some people are more resilient than others. Some traumatic events can be too severe for the autonomic nervous system to handle, and it will be unable to recover unaided.

We all have our own specific reaction to a traumatic event. No matter how shocking the event is, some people feel all they need to feel and express all they need to express. After that, they can move on as their autonomic nervous system recovers from the shock and intensity of the event. The recovery may not be quick or easy, but it is moderate for the average person and faster than some people.

Some people may not be that lucky. They remain in that moment, dwelling in it and reliving it form that day henceforth. Their illusion of reality has chattered, and they are forever changed by the event, not in the right way. The event keeps draining and affecting them long after it happened. This is a state of perpetual fight or flight mode.

The sympathetic nerves are activated after a traumatic event, but the parasympathetic nerves are unable to return the body to rest or digest mode. This doesn't mean that they have PTSD. It means that they "could" have PTSD or depression. The activation of the sympathetic nerves may lead to a perpetual fight or flight response. That is what causes PTSD. The sympathetic nerves could also lead to a withdrawal or shutdown response, which is depression. Depression puts the autonomous nervous system in chronic dorsal vagal mode.

These two are the most significant extreme reactions that the body has to trauma. Both reactions prevent the patient from properly integrating with society and mingling with friends and family. A person who has PTSD is also likely to exhibit symptoms of depression. It shows that PTSD is more complex and severe than a depression. The inability to interact with society leaves many people with PTSD lonely and isolated. They may become violent or suicidal. We are yet to find a proper solution to PTSD. The options out there include medication and therapy, but they are mostly designed to manage the situation.

Most people don't consider it for what PTSD is, and it is a twist of the reactions generated sympathetic by the sympathetic nerves (the fight or flight mode). Everyday stress moves the autonomous nervous system towards the fight or flight mode. PTSD is actually a chronic dorsal vagal mode. The autonomic nervous system drives the body to hopelessness, fear, and apathy, instead of fight or fear. This means you can't treat PTSD the same way you would treat other reactions of the sympathetic nerves, such as chronic stress. It would be counter-productive, and it may elevate the conditions of the patient.

Psychologists and other medical practitioners often focus on the traumatic event when treating PTSD. They don't usually study the

Patients' psychological fixation on the traumatic event. It is the memories that trigger a spell. Telling someone (definitely a professional) about the event may alleviate the impact of the condition. It could also backfire by triggering an episode. Recalling an intense event may send the person into a hypnotic trance. It stimulates the emotions and brings back even with vivid details.

The psychologist may try other techniques such as integrating different techniques and exercises in treating a patient and helping the patient integrate back into society.

PTSD and the Dorsal Branch

One of the best ways to treat PTSD is to target the dorsal branch state. Bring the patient out of that mode, and all may be well. This procedure is a gradual process that needs to be practiced until it becomes second nature.

The dorsal vagal mode is not just a psychological issue, and it is much more than that. The problem won't be solved by talk therapy alone. It is more a combination of a physical and psychological issue. That is why it is aptly called a psychophysiological problem. The treatment of these kinds of health conditions with medication and drugs such as antidepressants and other stimulants only arouses the autonomous nervous system. It triggers the patient to be optimistic by releasing feel-good chemicals into the bloodstream, but it doesn't solve the main issue, which is why drugs alone are not the answer. It doesn't make the patient want to reintegrate into society or feel true happiness and joy.

Understanding the relationship between the dorsal branches of the vagus nerve and its relationship with PTSD can help in the treatment of the disorder. It will help in the treatment of other psychophysiological disorders and also psychological disorders. The dorsal branches' activities on the visceral organs caused PTSD. It is a state that decreases patients' and their loved ones' ability to live their lives effectively and happily. The treatments we have today are very expensive and not exactly efficient. It is an improvement in the way PTSD used to be treated in the past, but we still have a long way to go before we can get it right. The next step in the journey involves the vagus nerve. It involves appropriately examining the relationship between the autonomous nervous system and PTSD and using our understanding of that relationship to treat the disorder. Why medications and pills have not been the answer it may be possible to bring a person suffering from PTSD to fully functional recovery and social integration through the manipulation of the autonomic nervous system, where the problem really is.

The Autonomic Nervous System and Depression

The population of the American public dealing with depression is baffling. Depression is now worse than obesity. Out of all the mental health conditions in the United States, about 10 percent is depression. American has turned to prescription churning out pills and handing them out to pretty much any of these depressed people. Antidepressants and related medications are the most prescribed and purchased medications. They account for a third of all the prescription drugs used in the United States. This problem is not just an American issue. The sales of antidepressants in 2013 raked in north of $9.8 billion.

The most obvious symptom of depression is a lack of interest. A person battling depression doesn't want to do anything, especially with other people. They are apathetic, inactive, unmotivated, lack appetite, or eat too much and many others.

Depression is about feelings, negative feelings. The negative emotions influence the person with depressive actions and habits. These are examples of the feelings that a depressed person has:

- Sadness

- Hopelessness

- Emptiness

- Shame

- Guilt

- Restlessness

- Anxiety

- Apathy

- Lethargy

- Lack of motivation

All of these emotions affect their memory and decision-making ability. They are unable to concentrate, and they may also experience pains and aches. Depression becomes extreme when the person starts self-harming or become suicidal. This is due to the sympathetic nerves' activities, which stimulate the autonomic nervous system into a chronic dorsal mode.

A medical caregiver such as a therapist or doctor will question you and monitor your reactions and responses, even your medical history before you can diagnose you as a depressant. The doctor won't consider that the situation is a state; he believes it is a temporary phase and prescribes some drugs. The medication works, but it is quick, and you have to take another one when it wears off. Then this becomes a daily thing, and you get on the medication, taking it every day for the next few weeks, months, or even years.

It becomes a thing until you become desensitized to the medication and try a stronger dosage or a different drug. Medicine doesn't really solve the problem it just helps you maintain it.

When you are already on medication, it is a terrible idea to stop taking a medication without the physician's consent, especially the physician who prescribed it, if you can find him. That's not to say you should stop taking medication; if you find a better option or feel it is working, you should seek an expert's opinion before making the decision and receive advice on the best way to proceed.

This is mostly due to withdrawal. Most medicines have a withdrawal effect on the body. When you have taken a medication for so long that your body is used to having it in your bloodstream, you need to wean the body away from that drug. If this is not done correctly, the body may react.

If the general public is not reading these credible sources of information, indeed, the doctors are. Yet they still prescribe antidepressants for anyone with a mild case of depressants. Sure, therapists still want you to undergo talk therapy, but when you complain about depression to your doctor, you are most likely to visit the pharmacy.

Why do doctors still prescribe antidepressants, or why do intelligent people who have access to the right information even ask for antidepressants?

The problem is similar to their treatments of PTSD. Most people, including doctors, do not fully understand the impact of the autonomous nervous system. It is the main issue in this case, and you have to affect it before you can treat depression. But antidepressants don't work on the autonomous nervous system because it is resilient and flexible. Any effect will be temporary because it will later adjust itself.

Medicine doesn't pay attention to the physiology of depression; most of the emphasis is on the physiology of chronic stress. Doctors don't focus on the dorsal branch activity of the vagus nerve and the autonomous nervous system.

That is where our study of the anatomy of the vagus nerve comes in. It exposes a new understanding of the central nervous system that most people didn't pay attention to before, and few are only beginning to consider. It shows that there are safe, efficient alternatives to our current techniques and processes for treating some diseases.

CONCLUSION

In conclusion, vagus nerve contributes to such a significant number of functions in our bodies, keeping it as "happy" as conceivably ought to be of prime significance. This doesn't imply that you need to stress over each easily overlooked detail you do, just as with each side effect that appears as though identified with vagus nerve damage. Instead, watch and partake in those things that relax you and whatever makes you happy. Evade excessive drinking and propensities that lead to diabetes or related ailments. As you deal with your vagus nerve, it most likely deals with you consequently.

Incessant pressure, or a steady pressure experienced over a drawn-out timeframe, can add to long haul issues for heart and veins. The constant and continuous increment in pulse, and the raised degrees of stress hormones and circulatory strain, can negatively affect the body. This continuous long-haul pressure can build a hazard for hypertension, coronary failure, or stroke.

Rehashed intense pressure and diligent interminable pressure may likewise add to irritation in the circulatory framework, especially in the coronary courses. This is one pathway that is thought to bind worry to cardiovascular failure. It likewise creates the impression of how an individual reacts to pressure can influence cholesterol levels.

The hazard for coronary illness related to pressure seems to vary for ladies, contingent upon whether the lady is pre or postmenopausal. Levels of estrogen in premenopausal ladies seem to help veins react better during pressure along these lines helping their bodies to all the more likely handle pressure and ensuring them against coronary illness. Postmenopausal ladies lose this degree of security because of loss of estrogen, along these lines putting them at more serious hazard for the impacts of weight on coronary illness.

Endocrine

When somebody sees a circumstance to be challenged, undermining or wild, the cerebrum starts a course of occasions including the hypothalamic-pituitary-adrenal (HPA) hub, which is the essential driver of the endocrine pressure reaction. This, finally, results in an expansion in the generation of steroid hormones called glucocorticoids, which incorporate cortisol, frequently alluded to as the "stress hormone."

The HPA hub

During times of pressure, the nerve center, a gathering of cores that interfaces the mind and the endocrine framework, flag the pituitary organ to deliver a hormone, which thus flags the adrenal organs, situated over the kidneys, to build the generation of cortisol. Cortisol expands the degree of vitality fuel accessible by assembling glucose and unsaturated fats from the liver. Cortisol is regularly created in fluctuating levels for the day, commonly growing in fixation after arousing and gradually declining for the day, giving a day by day cycle of vitality. An expansion in cortisol can furnish the vitality required to manage drawn-out or great tests during an unpleasant occasion.

Stress and wellbeing

Glucocorticoids, including cortisol, are significant for managing the invulnerable framework and diminishing irritation. While this is important during upsetting or undermining circumstances where damage may bring about expanded insusceptible framework enactment, constant pressure can get about impeded correspondence between the safe framework and the HPA pivot. This disabled correspondence has been connected to the future improvement of various physical and psychological wellbeing conditions, including constant exhaustion, metabolic issues (e.g., diabetes, obesity), discouragement, and safety issues.

Gastrointestinal

The gut has a massive number of neurons that can work reasonably freely and are in steady correspondence with the mind disclosing the capacity to feel "butterflies" in the stomach. Stress can influence this mind's gut correspondence and may trigger agony, swelling, and other gut inconvenience to be handled all the more effectively. The gut is likewise occupied by a great many microorganisms which can impact its wellbeing and the mind's wellbeing, which can affect the capacity to think and influence feelings. Stress is related to changes in gut microorganisms, which thus can impact the state of mind. Subsequently, the gut's nerves and microscopic organisms emphatically affect the mind and the other way around.

Early life stress can change the improvement of the sensory system just as how the body responds to pressure. These progressions can expand the hazard for later gut sicknesses or dysfunction.

In short words, the vagus nerve represents our most important nerve and due to its benefits, you had no idea that it exists up until now. If you start researching about it, you will also see that there is not that much information available. That is simply because the medical industry does not benefit from it and has to sell more and more medication.

It is connected to many organs and system in the body as we elaborated above and should be properly stimulated with the previously mentioned exercises. Those exercises will properly stimulate it and fix whatever problem you are facing with. Exercises for stimulating the vagus nerve are beneficial not only for your brain but also for your overall mental and physical health.

Last but most important, do not forget to laugh. Laughter is the best exercise and the best medicine against everything and stimulates the vagus nerve like no other exercise known.

Made in the USA
Las Vegas, NV
08 April 2022

47083191R00085